Education of Health Professionals in Complementary/Alternative Medicine

*A Conference Sponsored by the
Josiah Macy, Jr. Foundation*

Chaired by Alfred P. Fishman, M.D.

*Phoenix, Arizona
November 2-5, 2000*

Edited by Mary Hager

*Published by the
Josiah Macy, Jr. Foundation
44 East 64th Street
New York, NY 10021*

2001

Table of Contents

Editor's Note

In November 2000 the Josiah Macy, Jr. Foundation convened a conference that was designed to develop guidance for medical and health professional schools in the teaching about complementary and alternative medicine (CAM). Participants felt the conference was timely given the escalating phenomena of CAM usage by the public. Questions of definition, standardization, efficacy and appropriate usage were discussed. At the conclusion of the conference, participants developed and approved a consensus statement and a set of recommendations.

Preface

This volume is the product of a Macy Foundation conference on Complementary and Alternative Medicine that was held in Phoenix, AZ, in November 2000. The original idea for the conference was put forward by Dr. Alfred Fishman of the University of Pennsylvania, who argued persuasively that the topic was in urgent need of attention, and who agreed to serve as Chairman of the conference. The overall goal of the papers, discussions and deliberations was to identify appropriate responses on the part of educational institutions of the "traditional" (western) health professions in the United States to the high public demand for, and utilization of "non-traditional" therapies.

The planning committee debated about what term should be used to designate the overall topic. The use of the phrase "integrative medicine" was coming into increasing use at the time of those discussions, and it was agreed that there was much to recommend it as a blanket term of reference. However, the National Institutes of Health had named its relevant component the Office of Complementary and Alternative Medicine, and it was ultimately decided that, for purposes of easy identification, that official title should prevail. Thus the subject of this book is referred to throughout as Complementary and Alternative Medicine, or CAM.

Several papers were commissioned in advance of the conference and are represented herein. In addition, there were excellent presentations and discussion from conference participants, and an effort has been made to capture the substance and tone of those entries as well. As can be deduced from the list of participants, an effort was made to include a variety of voices from both traditional and CAM arenas, in order to achieve a reasoned and balanced discourse on topics that are often inflammatory. That goal was achieved to a remarkable extent during the conference itself, and it is hoped that some of the spirit of collegiality that prevailed during the meeting is captured in this volume.

An Executive Summary is presented at the outset, which provides an encapsulation of two- and one-half days of rich discussion; a statement of the principles on which recommendations were based; and then a set of recommendations to which the conferees agreed with amity and enthusiasm. Following that, individual chapters deal with the current status of CAM in medical and other health professional schools, with issues of the validity or need for scientific verification of various CAM modalities, and with the present-day realities of popular usage, access and cost of CAM in the United States. A few presentations approached the important issue of population diversity as it relates to CAM usage, but it was generally agreed that far too few data existed to inform that important discussion. Nevertheless, it is hoped that the reader can obtain a useful framework for further analysis of a highly complex and often murky set of issues pertinent both to traditional "western" medicine and to CAM, especially as they relate to the future education of health professionals.

What we hope can be found in this volume are useful answers to a series of timely questions. What is actually happening these days in the area of CAM, focusing on health professional education (generally medical education, although not exclusively)? What is it that should be taught, and what not? What should be done in terms of research that could validate or strengthen areas in which there appears to be promise but for which the data have not yet been developed? And what kinds of information sources could be created that could allow the medical profession, in particular, to be more literate in this area?

Having gone through those deliberations and recommendations, I am impressed that, if nothing else, we have been doing our students a great disservice by leaving them illiterate about a whole field of therapeutic or healing endeavors. Certainly something needs to be done. We need to consider who will do that teaching, how they should become adept at such instruction, and when and what referral patterns should be recommended to our students. If we can provide guidance to those on the front lines of health professional education about those fundamental issues, I believe we will have done both the American public and the health professions a significant service.

I am particularly grateful to Dr. Fishman for his strong leadership in this endeavor and to the planning committee members whose efforts are reflected in this monograph. On a sad and special note, I would like to pay particular tribute to one member of the planning committee, Alice Trillin. She played the challenging role of representing a "consumer voice" both during the planning process and then at the conference, and she greatly enriched our deliberations. While this book was in preparation, the delayed after-effects of her long-ago illness, and its therapy, which she discussed in her paper (*vide infra*) resurfaced and resulted in an inexorable series of setbacks, ultimately proving lethal. Alice had contributed professionally over the years to analysis of effective communication about health matters, to people of all ages but especially to children; and we were fortunate to be the beneficiaries of her insight and wisdom in this endeavor. It is with gratitude, therefore, that I acknowledge the special grace that she brought to our effort. We have reproduced her talk as she presented it to the conferees, without alteration, in the hopes that the reader can capture some of the wisdom and spirit she shared so generously.

As this monograph was in galley-proof stage, the sad news of Dr. Alvan Feinstein's death also reached us. His remarkable contributions to American Medicine were widely recognized, and his participation in our conference lent it special distinction. I am particularly proud that his important paper on the placebo effect constitutes one of the major contributions of the conference, and that he had been able to take the time to update it in light of subsequent published discussions about placebos (see p. 89).

June E. Osborn MD

June E. Osborn, M.D.

President, Josiah Macy, Jr. Foundation

In Memoriam

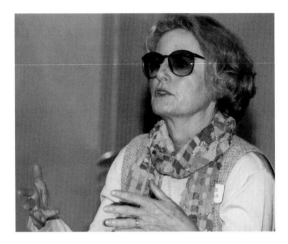

Alice Trillin 1939 - 2001

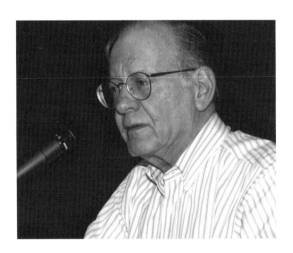

Alvan Feinstein 1925 - 2001

Introduction

Alternative Medicine in the Academic Medical Center

Alfred P. Fishman, M.D.
University of Pennsylvania School of Medicine

Chairman

Academic medical centers are currently facing up to the challenge of incorporating so-called "Alternative Medicine" into the educational programs of their scientifically-based institutions. No longer is the question "should it be done?" Instead, the question is "how to do it?" This meeting was devoted to some of the issues that have to be addressed in order to take full advantage of that prospect. Among the barriers to be overcome are the over crowded medical curriculum, ambiguities in nomenclature, the unsettled contemporary medical scene, and mutual misunderstanding.

The Overcrowded Medical Curriculum

The typical curriculum is a conglomerate which is already bulging at the seams with the triumphs of scientific medicine. Simply adding courses is neither feasible nor desirable. Integration holds more promise for meaningful incorporation of alternative medicine into the medical curriculum than does addition. However, the process of integration requires understanding and accommodation by clinical scientists who are apt to be reluctant to make way for therapies which they regard as unconventional and unproven.

Nomenclature

Ambiguity in terminology not only hampers communication but also compromises research and education. For medical educators, the designation "Alternative Medicine" entails the threat of displacing conventional medicine for the sake of unproven therapies from other medical traditions. Moreover, although "Alternative Medicine" covers a panoply of diverse therapies, it lacks the organization and processes of scientific medicine. The disparities relate to the call for integration of unconventional therapies into western medicine.

Integration is not a simple process for unmatched systems. The lead definition in Webster's New World College Dictionary characterizes the process as "to make whole or complete by adding or bringing together parts." Although unconventional therapies share many beliefs as common denominators, such as vitalism, the healing power of nature and spiritual mind-body interplay, the lack of organized structure and process dictates that each unconventional modality be incorporated separately into western medicine.

As a practical expedient, the term "Complementary" has become popular currency. The term signifies that a given therapy borrowed from another culture is an addition to, or an enhancement of, western medical therapy and not a substitute (Table 1). As a corollary, once safety and efficacy are proven by western criteria, complementary therapies become part of conventional medicine.

Even more pervasive than "Complementary" has become the abbreviation "CAM. Originally a by-product of the creation of a center at the National Institutes of Health for "Complementary/Alternative Medicine," the abbreviation has become commonplace, more often used as a synonym for a complementary than for an alternative therapy.

The Unsettled Contemporary Medical Scene

Few would challenge that contemporary medicine is restless and undergoing dramatic change. Forces outside of medicine are shaping the practice of medicine while physicians, educated to deliver acute care, face novel demands imposed by the need for chronic care, unanticipated epidemics and increasingly diverse populations. Meanwhile, scientific medicine and technologic advance are in high gear, rapidly generating new, albeit expensive, diagnostic methods and therapies.

In this unsteady state, how can the education of the physician with respect to complementary therapies contribute to the care of the patient? This question was probed by the meeting that is the basis for this book.

Mutual Misunderstanding

Health care practitioners of unconventional therapies are usually unfamiliar with the principles and practice of scientific medicine, just as practitioners of conventional medicine rarely have insights into the cultures and beliefs of those who practice unconventional therapies. Many of the latter are not physicians. Of the two deficiencies, the more readily remediable seems to be an increase in the appreciation of cultural diversity by western physicians. This insight would promise not only better utilization of therapies derived from other traditions, but also better interplay with patients from diverse backgrounds. Less corrigible for the immediate future is the lack of research training by health professionals who practice unconventional therapies. A sample of a scientific approach is shown in Table 2. Attention and elimination of misunderstanding by both sides seems to be prerequisite for the incorporation of complementary therapies into western medicine.

The Scope and Sequence of the Meeting

The meeting sponsored by the Josiah Macy, Jr. Foundation that constitutes the substrate for this book addressed the question of education in complementary medicine with particular reference to barriers that had to be overcome in order for complementary therapies to be incorporated into the conventional medical curriculum.

To set the stage, five position papers were invited for pre-circulation among the participants. These were intended to provide background and content for discussion subsequently by the participants. At the meeting, the oral presentations began with brief surveys of how some academic medical centers are dealing with complementary therapies, followed by consideration of general issues that have to be taken into account in planning for incorporating complementary therapies into medical education. An animated discussion, especially by educators and practitioners of unconventional medicine, urged integration of complementary therapies into conventional medical education while challenging the hegemony of scientific medicine. In turn, academic medical voices seconded the need for awareness of CAM on the part of medical students and practitioners of western health care, but underscored the need for evidence to justify implementation of therapies in standard care.

Participants at the Conference

Alfred P. Fishman, M.D. *
University of Pennsylvania
Medical School
Chair

Dyanne D. Affonso, Ph.D., R.N.*
University of Nebraska

Lenore Arab, Ph.D.
University of North Carolina
at Chapel Hill

Wade M. Aubry, M.D.
The Lewin Group

Brian M. Berman, M.D.
University of Maryland

Roger J. Bulger, M.D.
Association of Academic Health
Centers

Ruth Ellen Bulger, Ph.D.
Uniformed Services University
of the Health Sciences

Harvey R. Colten, M.D.
iMetrikus, Inc.

Richard A. Cooper, M.D.
Medical College of Wisconsin

David M. Eisenberg, M.D.
Beth Israel Deaconess Medical
Center

Leon Eisenberg, M.D.*
Harvard Medical School

Alvan R. Feinstein, M.D.
Yale University School of Medicine

Charles K. Francis, M.D.
Charles R. Drew University of Medicine
and Science

Tracy W. Gaudet, M.D.
Duke University Medical Center

**Kim A. Jobst, M.A., D.M., M.R.C.P.,
M.F.Hom.**
Oxford Brookes University

Wayne B. Jonas, M.D.*
Uniformed Services University of the
Health Sciences

Harry R. Kimball, M.D., M.A.C.P.
American Board of Internal Medicine

Aaron Lazare, M.D.
University of Massachusetts
at Worcester

Marc S. Micozzi, M.D., Ph.D.*
The College of Physicians
of Philadelphia

Bonnie O'Connor, Ph.D.
Hasbro Children's Hospital
Providence, RI

Karen N. Olness, M.D.
Case Western Reserve University

Herbert Pardes, M.D.
Columbia University

Reed Phillips, D.C., Ph.D.
Southern California University of
Health Sciences

Joseph E. Pizzorno, Jr., N.D.
Bastyr University

Carolyn B. Robinowitz, M.D.
Georgetown University

Robert M. Rose, M.D.
MacArthur Foundation

Peter V. Scoles, M.D.
National Board of Examiners

Brian L. Strom, M.D., M.P.H.*
University of Pennsylvania

Alice Stewart Trillin*
Consumer/Consultant

Miriam Wetzel, Ph.D.
Harvard Medical School

Michael E. Whitcomb, M.D.
Association of American Medical
Colleges

Lisa Corbin Winslow, M.D.
University of Colorado Health Sciences
Center

**MACY FOUNDATON
BOARD ATTENDEES**

Clarence Michalis

Harold Amos, Ph.D.

Bernard Harleston, Ph.D.

Arthur H. Hayes, Jr., M.D.

June E. Osborn, M.D.

STAFF

Martha Wolfgang, M.S.W., M.P.H.

Tanya Tyler

Tashi Dakar Ridley

Mary Hager

* Planning Committee

Conference Attendees

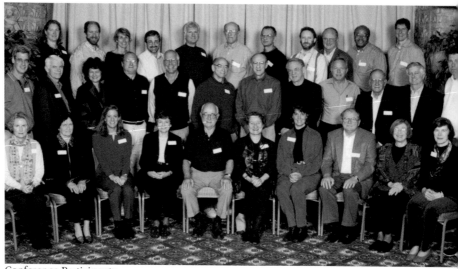

Conference Participants

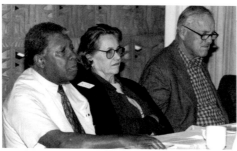

Harold Amos, Ph.D. (Board member)
Cora Michalis, Clarence Michalis (Board member)

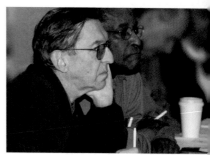

Arthur Hayes M.D., (Board member),
Bernard Harleston, Ph.D. (Board member)

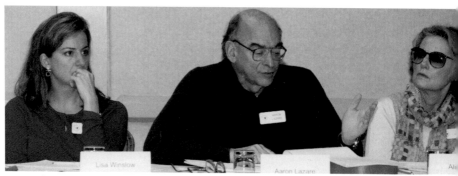

Lisa Corbin Winslow, M.D., Aaron Lazare, M.D., and Alice Stewart Trillin

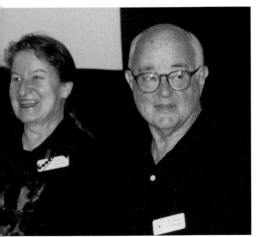

E. Osborn, M.D., President of the Macy Foundation
lfred P. Fishman, M.D., Conference Chairman

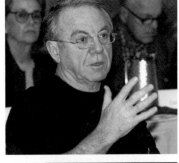

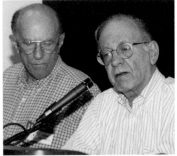

top right:
Herbert Pardes, M.D.

center right:
Leon Eisenberg M.D. and
Alvan Feinstein M.D.

bottom right:
Charles Francis, M.D.

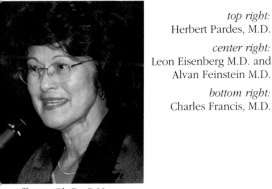

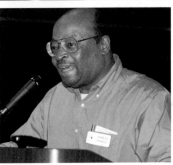

ne Affonso, Ph.D., R.N.

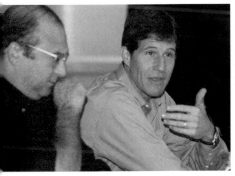

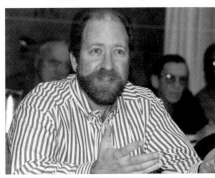

S. Micozzi, M.D., Ph.D.* and Wayne B. Jonas, M.D.   David Eisenberg, M.D.

15

Executive Summary
of the Conference

Recent surveys show that at least half of the population in the United States uses one of the diverse array of complementary and alternative medicine practices now known collectively by the acronym CAM. Virtually all of these are complementary rather than alternative. That use has grown dramatically over the past decades despite the fact that few insurance plans provide coverage for any of the many CAM procedures. Users pay an estimated $27 billion a year out of pocket for these services and make more visits to CAM providers than to primary care physicians.

As another indication of how firmly entrenched in the health care system CAM has become, the National Center for Complementary/Alternative Medicine at the National Institutes of Health invests more than $50 million a year to investigate the safety and efficacy of some of these approaches. Too, such well-known institutions as Memorial Sloan Kettering Cancer Center and a small, but growing, number of health maintenance organizations and insurance plans now offer some CAM procedures. Nor has big business ignored the growing appeal of CAM, for herbal remedies, alone, have become a $10 billion a year industry that is growing at a projected annual rate of 20-30 percent.

No single definition adequately captures the range of practices that fall under the CAM rubric. Even those that simply define CAM as practices that are not part of mainstream medicine, or as practices used by patients to manage their own health care, or as therapies that are not widely taught in western medical schools or available in most hospitals, fail to capture the complexity of the field. CAM includes health care practices that range from the use of vitamins, herbal remedies and massage therapies to the ancient traditions of Ayurveda and Chinese medicine, along with chiropractic, naturopathy, homeopathic medicine, meditation, hypnosis, acupuncture and a host of other lesser known approaches to health and health care.

Though their use is common and standard practice in much of the world, most CAM procedures have never been tested according to the rigorous, scientific standards of western, evidence-based medicine. Because of this, the response of medical practitioners to the growing CAM phenomenon has ranged from an outright dismissal of practices not proven safe and effective to a gradual recognition that such extensive use can no longer be ignored. Several surveys suggest that at least half of practicing physicians want to know more about CAM so they can advise and guide their patients.

Other studies show that most CAM users are not abandoning western medicine but want the best of both worlds – an alternative caregiver with strong ties to the medical establishment and a physician who both understands and will make appropriate referrals for CAM therapies. But this poses yet another problem for physicians, for studies also show that many CAM users do not tell their physicians what they are doing and that most practicing physicians know almost nothing about the potential benefits or risks of CAM because their training has focused almost exclusively on western scientific medicine.

Academic health centers have started to respond to the challenge of CAM, both by introducing content into medical curricula and by considering research on some of these approaches, perhaps because they recognize that by ignoring CAM, they will fail future physicians and their patients. Yet questions abound, for it is far from clear how teaching institutions should address what has, in effect, become a parallel system of health care. What should they teach and who should do the teaching? What research needs to be done, and for which CAM approaches? And how should teaching institutions insert this admittedly controversial material into already crowded curricula?

Macy Conference addresses questions

With its long-standing commitment to the education of health professionals, the Josiah Macy, Jr. Foundation convened a conference in November of 2000 to examine such questions. The conference, "Education of Health Professionals in Complementary/Alternative Medicine," brought together consumers, CAM and mainstream practitioners, medical school deans, and physicians and other health care professionals who have experience with CAM and have looked for ways to integrate these approaches into a mainstream medical education program. Alfred P. Fishman, M.D., Senior Associate Dean for Program Development at the University of Pennsylvania Medical School, served as chair.

Presentations and discussions at the two- and a half-day conference explored the challenges to medical education posed by CAM from many directions, including a brief look at the history and ancient roots of traditional practices, the research that has been done to establish the safety and efficacy of some of these approaches, and the role of multiculturalism in the use of these therapies. At the end of the conference, participants agreed on the brief consensus statement and set of recommendations found at the end of this summary.

CAM is a government-inspired acronym that has become accepted shorthand in the U.S. for what is known as integrative medicine in much of Europe and much of which is considered mainstream medicine in many parts of the world. From the beginning of the conference, it was not clear how participants could find sufficient common ground to deal with the diverse array of practices that fall under the CAM rubric.

The appeal of CAM

What was clear, though, was that many CAM therapies are widely used by the public, even though they fail to meet the standards of evidence-based medicine. Still, to many at the conference the reasons for CAM's popularity was clear. CAM practitioners spend time with patients, an average of 30 minutes per session, whereas under managed care, physicians today spend an average of seven minutes. As one participant observed, the real issue is not whether the appeal of CAM relies on anecdote or science but that western medicine, bowing to financial pressures and the ease of handing out pills, increasingly ignores both the patient and the patient's context.

Another appeal comes from the fact that most CAM approaches are rooted in the belief that health is not determined by a given medical system or tradition but involves the interaction of mind and body. Practices tend to focus on healing and therapies that are aimed at maintenance of health, not illness and disease. Touch, caring and healing are essential ingredients and many CAM practices stress the importance of self-care and the beliefs and attitudes that influence healing. CAM systems tend to emphasize the individual and work with natural processes. They are therapeutically conservative and value knowledge and wisdom gained through experience. Participants were reminded of the sharp philosophical differences between CAM and mainstream medicine. Unlike many CAM approaches, medicine today deals with illness and disease, focusing on isolated body systems, not on the whole body or mind-body interactions. Treatments are based on therapeutic activism and an effort to dominate natural processes, with high value placed on technological knowledge and skills, and standardized approaches.

The broad usage of CAM

While its growth has coincided with both the rise of multiculturalism and greater affluence, the appeal of CAM seems far broader, for the use of CAM therapies is not confined to any one segment of the population. According to recent surveys, use is slightly higher among women than men, slightly lower among African Americans, and slightly higher on the west coast. Use is also slightly higher among those with more education and in the higher income brackets. These surveys also show that use cuts across age and economic barriers. "Baby boomers" are frequent users, more for prevention and lifestyle than therapeutic intervention; those under 30 in "generation X" are even more frequent users, again for lifestyle. At the same time, nearly one third of those over 65 have used at least one CAM intervention to treat a serious illness and about 20 percent have visited a CAM provider. And, though few CAM therapies are covered by any form of insurance, some 43 percent of people making less than $20,000 a year spend at least $250 annually for this kind of help.

Little information exists about use of CAM approaches among minority populations. What data do exist suggest that use patterns are very different, and that use is increasing. One study of Latino, black, white and Chinese women with breast cancer showed at least half had used one alternative approach and one third had used two. Yet use differed along racial and ethnic lines. Blacks turned more to spiritual healing, Chinese to herbal remedies, the Latino women to dietary and spiritual approaches and the whites to dietary and physical therapies like massage and acupuncture. Such differences, though, cloud the fact of heterogeneity within cultural and ethnic groups and ignore variations in use patterns in different parts of the country.

Because so many people are reluctant to admit to CAM use, existing studies underestimate the extent of CAM use, participants were reminded. These studies show that half of the estimated 600 million annual visits to CAM practitioners are for massage and chiropractic procedures and that at least 10 percent of the population admits to using chiropractic, massage, herbal remedies, relaxation and meditation techniques.

And they are willing to pay for perceived benefits. People spend an estimated $27 to 34 billion every year for techniques that include chiropractic, acupuncture and massage, biofeedback, megavitamins, homeopathy, relaxation and meditation, spiritual healing, folk remedies, lifestyle diets, herbal remedies and energy healing. Some CAM practices are no longer considered unorthodox, having been accepted by mainstream medicine as complementary therapies. An NIH consensus conference approved the use of acupuncture for certain types of pain, while federal guidelines recommend chiropractic techniques for low back pain. Psychosocial support for cancer patients is well established in many institutions. Even health maintenance organizations are starting to offer some CAM therapies for their patients though greater coverage has been slowed by worries about the broader implications of establishing a precedent for paying for unproven, experimental therapies.

Patients' reluctance to discuss CAM use

As lines between mainstream medicine and CAM have blurred, surveys show patients are still reluctant to discuss their use of complementary approaches with their physicians. Even though 97 percent of CAM users also have a regular physician, more than 60 percent don't tell their physicians about their involvement with CAM — either because physicians don't ask or because patients don't feel comfortable telling their physicians that they use other therapies.

Participants explored reasons behind this communication failure, wondering about the role shame and humiliation may play. Physicians are shame-prone; humiliation is part of their training and they are particularly humiliated by HMOs and even the threat of malpractice. Patients, in turn, are ashamed to tell doctors why they seek unconventional therapies, when they go to other physicians, even what kinds of medicine they are taking.

This communication failure has a negative impact on health and patient care. It erodes trust, which is fundamental to a good doctor-patient relationship. But failure to communicate can also lead to serious complications. Physicians need to know about the use of herbs that interact with prescribed medications or exert direct toxic effects.

Such potential problems underpin the demands of many in mainstream medicine that CAM therapies be tested for safety and efficacy through the same type of clinical trials required for mainstream therapies — even though, as one participant reminded, at least 85 percent of what western medicine does has never been subjected to this kind of scrutiny and a recent Institute of Medicine study documented an alarming number of deaths due to mistakes and inappropriate use of approved medications.

These demands by mainstream medicine would ignore anecdotal evidence and personal experience, which guide much use of CAM therapies, in favor of controlled scientific studies with results published in peer-reviewed journals and replicated by other researchers. They also insist that vitamins, herbs and other CAM remedies be subjected to the same federal approval mechanisms required for pharmaceutical agents. Under current law, such remedies are considered food supplements which require no advance approval by the Food and Drug Administration. Federal regulation is needed if only to ensure that dosages are standardized and products meet some kind of quality guidelines.

Directions for future research

While CAM participants at the meeting supported the call for more research, they also pointed out that many procedures can never meet the "gold-standard" of a double-blind, controlled clinical trial which seeks to isolate a single, effective agent. Many CAM approaches used in western societies, they pointed out, are integral in the original medical tradition, to an entire system of care. Even the trials that have documented the effectiveness of acupuncture for certain problems ignored the "whole-system approach," nor have the results achieved by experienced practitioners been taken into full account. Further, they observed, manufacturers of vitamin and herbal supplements that are already widely available have no incentive to spend the millions of dollars required for clinical trials.

Many CAM practices also defy conventional scientific testing because they deal with chronic, subjective and individualized complaints difficult to measure precisely. Some participants noted

21

that rigid scientific studies ignore such vital but often untestable contributions to therapeutic effectiveness as the "bedside manner" of the practitioner, the spontaneous healing forces of nature, the expectations of the patient, and the therapeutic response that comes from any therapy, elements often grouped as the "placebo effect." For some patients, it was pointed out the placebo effect is so powerful that even the decision to seek help seems to provide relief.

From their discussions, participants seemed to agree that science-based medicine and CAM can learn from each other. For instance, medical practitioners could help patients by learning when to use effective CAM therapies for such chronic conditions as low back pain; conversely CAM providers need to recognize when to refer for medical care patients with conditions for whom orthodox therapy might be curative or life-saving: meningitis was offered as an example. Medical practitioners might benefit by learning to make better use of the placebo effect and natural forces of healing, and by returning to a time when patient therapy was provided with far more attention to caring than curing, several participants commented.

At the same time, participants agreed that more research was needed to assess the safety and effectiveness of various CAM therapies. Both CAM and orthodox providers need to help the public overcome the belief that "natural equals safe" or that a preparation is safe simply because it has been used for thousands of years, especially since it is not clear precisely what ingredients some of these remedies contain. Lack of standardization has made it difficult, if not impossible, to test some of these remedies. Chemical analysis in one prospective study, for instance, revealed that a preparation to be tested contained none of the reported active ingredient.

Because CAM covers such a wide and diverse group of approaches to health and health care, many participants supported an approach to further research that would group therapies into those which demanded further testing for safety and efficacy, those which were probably safe, and those with a higher risk in which any use should be dissuaded. CAM providers could provide a useful service by giving a straightforward account of what conditions were treated and keeping track of outcomes, they suggested. Such information would help physicians guide their patients to the use of CAM practices that are safe and may be beneficial and to dissuade them from using those practices with a greater risk of being unsafe.

The teaching dilemma

The question of what and how to teach medical students proved difficult to answer. While the explosion of interest in CAM therapies requires that physicians need to know what patients are using and the potential problem areas, and also where to find reliable information to guide their patients, participants agreed physicians do not need to become competent in delivering CAM therapies. They do, however, need to know when, where and how to refer their patients. Because of financial pressures and already crowded curricula, participants agreed that any effort to introduce formal courses addressing CAM would be unworkable. They also agreed that teaching physicians to be CAM practitioners would be both impractical and unnecessary, and acknowledged that each institution would have to design its own strategies for teaching CAM.

Based on their own experiences integrating CAM approaches into a medical curriculum, several participants emphasized the need to teach students the art of communicating with and listening to patients. Having medical students actually experience some of these approaches has proven effective. In one program, for instance, students were hooked to a biofeedback device to experience how they could change physiological parameters by changing their thinking, or were taught yoga and meditation. The experience effectively changed the way the students viewed alternative approaches and also improved the way they interacted with patients. Other programs have emphasized self-care for students.

In terms of who should do the teaching, those with experience in the field suggested that CAM practitioners be involved since few physicians have sufficient knowledge to teach about CAM. Also, as participants were reminded, definitions of health, illness and appropriate care differ by culture, religious and philosophical beliefs. Therefore, students need to be exposed to and taught about these differences in definition and beliefs.

Concluding Statements

At the conclusion of their deliberations, participants agreed upon the following concluding statements and recommendations:

- More Americans visit CAM practitioners in a given week than consult primary care practitioners. Most of these CAM clients also see their physicians but only a minority share that information with their physicians, unaware of the risks of untoward interactions between the two systems of care or of what benefits might be expected from CAM approaches.

- Most physicians are unfamiliar with the theories and practice of CAM and the extent of their patients' adherence to those approaches. Therefore, the education of medical students, as well as resident and practicing physicians, must include sufficient information about the theories and practices of CAM approaches to permit them to provide more comprehensive care for their patients.

- Efforts to expand knowledge about CAM should extend beyond the education of medical students. The education of all health professionals should include familiarity with CAM practices, as well as what is known about the efficacy of various CAM practices and the potential risks and benefits from the use of these practices.

Principles Underlying the Recommendations:

After deciding to limit the number of recommendations, participants emphasized the need to avoid any recommendations that would sound as if the group were either legitimizing CAM or reforming medicine. Their comments concerning the ingredients of recommendations took into account the following:

— Recommendations need to recognize that educating medical students about CAM is already taking place in most medical centers. To do this properly, the need for communicating risk/benefit and efficacy of common CAM procedures needs to be stressed. Licensure and research are essential ingredients as foundations for the teaching of medical students.

— Recommendations have to recognize that patients often seek CAM because they are looking for communication, compassion and hope. They also have to face up to the reality that physicians are now limited in the amount of time available for each patient. Is there a way around this dilemma?

— Recommendations should take into account that without proper reservations and qualifications, promoting efforts to communicate information about CAM to consumers may sound like a public relations promotion for CAM put out by the orthodox establishment. Communications to consumers also run the risk of attributing to a CAM modality the healing effect of personal interaction with a caring physician.

— Recommendations have to be based on an awareness that CAM practices can not be lumped together since CAM is not a single, homogenous entity but involves all kinds of practices with different levels of effectiveness and certainty. The focus, instead, should be to develop awareness of what is known and what is uncertain about CAM practices. Such an awareness is currently lacking in the orthodox medical community and in the patients who resort to these therapies.

— Recommendations have to address the question of how the public can be assured that CAM practitioners are competent. Along this line, standards have to be adopted for licensing and credentialling.

— Recommendations concerning CAM practices need to be considered within the context of the Surgeon General's goals for health promotion and disease prevention. Information about the best techniques for health promotion and disease prevention needs to be communicated by those practising CAM modalities as well as by medical practitioners.

— Recommendations should urge that medical physicians need to understand CAM and what CAM providers do so they can ensure the safety of their patients and set up procedures for appropriate referrals. There also is a need to assess the education of CAM providers, their practices and licensing requirements, to help CAM providers recognize when a medical referral is appropriate and to develop referral pathways and controls.

Recommendations

— Schools of medicine, nursing and pharmacy and academic health centers should integrate an awareness and knowledge of the most commonly used CAM theories and practices, with their potential for benefit and harm, as part of their curricula.

— Academic health centers should engage in rigorous collaborative, scientific research on the safety, efficacy and mechanisms of

CAM, involving those with expertise in CAM practices in these research efforts.

— Academic health centers should also initiate the collection of data about the use of CAM therapies and approaches in diverse cultural and ethnic settings.

— Professional and educational health care associations should make high quality, evidence-based CAM information widely available, include it in continuing education programs and encourage the provision of this high-quality information on the Internet and to the public.

— Professional licensing and credentialing bodies should include information pertinent to safety and efficacy of CAM procedures among their requirements.

Section I
Background

State of the Art

Alfred P. Fishman, M.D.

In 1993, western medicine had a rude awakening. A report in a prominent medical journal indicated that more than 40% of the American population was resorting to unconventional and unproven therapies.[11,44,48] By 1998, the situation had grown worse.[10,3,44] Some comfort could be taken from the fact that these deviants usually continued their standard medical care, i.e. the unconventional therapies were complementary rather than alternative. But, counterbalancing this reassurance was the news that few were telling their regular physicians about adding unconventional therapies to their medical management.

How to account for this unanticipated turnabout?[9,28,34] The idea of patients resorting to unproven therapies in the golden era of scientific medicine was mind-boggling. Never mind that not all therapies in western medicine had been proved to be scientifically sound. But as far as one could tell, the unproved conventional therapies were in keeping with the principles of scientific medicine, and sooner or later, these untested therapies would have to pass scientific scrutiny. Western medicine, as part of a social system, had to face up to the disquieting popular demand for unproven therapies.

Explanations for the surprising phenomenon came from different sources and directions.[24] One source implicated the decrease in patient-physician contact time imposed by managed care. Another saw the use of unconventional therapies as part of a general tendency for individuals to take greater control of their own lives.[6] A third pointed the finger at the ever-increasing reliance of physicians on high technology and the "dehumanization of medicine." Others pictured the physician as overly committed to curing rather than to caring. Some invoked all of the above and added a few of their own.

Physicians and academic institutions responded in various ways. Some physicians and clinics simply added unconventional modalities to their practices after reassuring themselves that these time-honored modalities promised to do no harm and might be helpful, either by some direct effect or as a placebo. Academic institutions faced more formidable obstacles: for example, how to reconcile their commitment to scientific medicine and the increasing call for evidence-based practice with the popular turn to unconventional and unproven remedies.[37,47,49,53,55] Was it ethical for physicians to refer patients for unproven remedies? Were there proper guidelines for credentialing?

Individual practitioners and academic institutions improvised. The federal government stepped in and created an office, followed by a center, the National Center for Complementary/Alternative Medicine, that would, in the tradition of the National Institutes of Health, sponsor research into the safety and efficacy of unproven remedies.[57]

Patterns of Response

The reflex response of academic institutions to the burgeoning popular demand for complementary therapies was denial: they refused to be swayed by the public uprising and simply reaffirmed allegiance to scientific and evidence-based medicine. But gradually, in keeping with the academic tradition of open-mindedness and receptivity of new ideas, an increasing number of academic medical centers began to take stock of how complementary therapies might relate to their missions in education, research and practice. By 1998, two-thirds of the academic medical centers offered some form of education about unconventional therapies. Usually the response was in the form of a single course: of these, 68% were isolated electives, 31% were part of required courses and 1% was part of an elective. Graduate medical education was less well-structured and far from uniform. Initiatives in research and education varied from institution to institution.

Organizations devoted to medical education soon recognized that organized medicine had to respond to the popular demand.[7,40] The Association of American Medical Colleges (AAMC) pointed out that physicians must be "sufficiently knowledgeable about both traditional and non-traditional modes of care to provide intelligent guidance to their patients."[39] The Society of Teachers of Family Medicine set forth recommendations for residency training that deal with attitudes, knowledge and skills concerning unconventional therapies. Included among the recommendations are provision for the development of understanding and respect for the basic theory or philosophy of the principal complementary/alternative treatment modalities, appreciation of the cultural influences on health beliefs, choices and practices, identification of the indications for such treatments, critical appraisal of the evidence for efficacy and cost-effectiveness of each modality, and awareness of the possible adverse effects of each modality. In addition, knowledge had to be gained of the positive as well as the negative effects of unconventional therapies.

The Case for Scientific Medicine

Systems for the delivery of health care are imbedded in the socio-economic fabric of western society. In this society, the physician has evolved as the icon of safe and effective medical practice. This preeminence has been assigned to the physician because he/she has undergone standardized medical education which is rooted in science.

Scientific medicine is a construct of concepts, data, facts, laws and procedures that has evolved over several centuries. It consists of two essential elements: content and process. The process determines how new knowledge materializes; the content is the product of the process. The content is the more variable of the two and changes as fresh insights and new understanding replace out-moded or erroneous knowledge. In contrast, the process which determines how new knowledge is acquired remains relatively fixed until a scientific revolution creates a new paradigm.[46] The process that determines the content of science is known as the scientific method. Modern medicine relies heavily on the scientific method, changing its content while the process is permanent. Not all that is currently practiced under the mantle of "scientific medicine" satisfies the requirements of scientific medicine. These untested practices have either been "grandfathered" into contemporary medical practice or are supported by empirical evidence of safety and efficacy.

Reproducibility is the cornerstone of scientific medicine and peer-reviewed journals represent the proving ground. Inevitably, once efficacy or safety of a practice becomes suspect, tests of reproducibility are begun. This self-cleansing process continually readjusts the content of scientific medicine.

Although scientific medicine is tuned to progress in science and technology, it remains rooted in Hippocratic tradition. This tradition dictates due regard for the patient and patient's rights, unremitting concern for the patients' welfare, painstaking observation and history-taking as key elements of proper practice. Above all, it includes respect for the Hippocratic admonition to "do no harm".

Shortcomings of Scientific Medicine

Criticisms of scientific medicine are often levied on the grounds of over reliance on mechanistic modalities with little regard for the interplay between mind, spirit and body. Increasingly, as new methods become available, this interplay is being addressed (see subsequent section). However, although modern medicine does rely heavily on its scientific bases, on evidence-based standards for practice and on mechanistic approaches to diagnosis, prevention and treatment, it would be blind-sighted to ignore its traditional focus on the patient-doctor relationship, respect for patient beliefs, and high regard for the humane and humanistic aspects of the care of the sick.

A more cogent criticism may be inadequate appreciation of the role of cultural diversity in determining the efficacy of health care.[23,41] The present meeting highlights this deficiency. It stresses, as will be apparent in the Discussion, that due regard is needed by the physician for the beliefs and practices of other cultures, including awareness of cultural approaches to health care that rely on concepts of vital forces and spirituality.[17] These topics were not specifically addressed at this meeting because each warrants more time than this meeting could provide.

Unfortunately, a variety of societal and financial pressures are putting implementation of the Hippocratic tradition into modern medical practice under considerable strain. For example, contact time between patient and physician has been abbreviated. Adverse events during hospitalization have shaken public confidence in western scientific medicine as the guarantor of patient safety. Accusations have been leveled that the physician has become overly reliant on high-technology and is more concerned with cure than with care. Ethical issues in the conduct of human research have made disquieting headlines. In response, the public, buttressed by an emerging populist movement, has turned in increasing numbers to another Hippocratic tradition, i.e. reliance on natural healing. In doing so, individuals are becoming better educated about health and healthy life-styles and are taking increasing responsibility for their own heath care.

The Case for Complementary Medicine

No matter how the unconventional therapies are labeled, i.e. "complementary," "alternative," "integrative," "natural," etc., they are not easily definable since they lack both the structure and the process that characterize "scientific medicine".[2] As a consequence, there is no question of incorporating complementary medicine as a generic entity into scientific medicine. Instead, each modality under the designation "complementary" will have to be assessed separately according to the process of scientific medicine. Fortunately, taken one-by-one, complementary therapies lend themselves to this process.[22]

The idea that culturally derived therapies may not be testable by the criteria of western scientific medicine has often been advanced by health professionals other than physicians. At first blush, this argument may be difficult to discount. Admittedly, beliefs and unseen forces can be difficult to quantify. However, there is neither mystery nor unreasonable complexity in applying the scientific method and advocates of unconventional therapies have to face the reality that it is unlikely that complementary therapies will be included in conventional medical armamentarium until they satisfy western standards.[42,47] Predictably, the tests will include reproducibility of safety, efficacy and cost-effectiveness. Obviously, once the tests have been passed, a complementary therapy can be incorporated into the fabric of conventional western scientific medicine.

Risk-Benefit-Cost Effectiveness

The span of Complementary/Alternative Medicine (CAM) consists of an array of therapies, which vary greatly in safety, efficacy and cost-effectiveness. Some, at one extreme, are harmless and require no elaborate studies to establish safety. At the other extreme are others, such as the use of acupuncture for asthma, which are intrinsically more hazardous.[36] The latter call for assessment of benefit vs. risk.

Not all complementary therapies require controlled clinical trials to satisfy standards for evidence-based medicine. Some such evidence already exists in the Cochrane Database of Systematic Reviews[14]. In 2000, the Cochrane collection included about 50 reviews of unconventional therapies and found that most of the evidence for their use to be inconclusive.[52] Nor are other critical reviews, such as those in the ACP Journal Club and in the journal *Evidence-Based Medicine*, more convincing. Part of the difficulty in evaluation is that trials have often been complicated by the simultaneous use of several modalities tailored to the perceived needs of the patient.

However this picture may be changing. For example, NIH-sponsored, controlled clinical trials are looking into whether St. John's Wort is useful in treating mild to moderate depression[50]. Another trial is doing the same for the saw palmetto treatment of benign prostatic hyperplasia.[56] A recent NIH consensus conference has endorsed the effectiveness of certain usages of acupuncture, as for low back pain and nausea.

Unfortunately, along with these promising prospects have come an increasing number of reports of adverse effects, particularly of harmful interactions between herbal remedies and prescribed medications.[12,43] Often it is difficult to decide whether dosage of the effective component or undiscovered components of the herbs are at fault. The uncertainties not only preclude generalizations about safety and efficacy but compromise research into mechanisms of action and role in health care.

A working group at the University of Pennsylvania, under the leadership of Dr. Brian Strom, undertook to draw distinctions between the options of individual practitioners with respect to the use of unconventional therapies and those of medical institutions which require guidelines and regulations to govern practice. For example, a physician who is caring for a patient who has taken a particular herb for a long while without side effects, has the option of condoning continued usage of the herbs on the basis of the patient's history and state of health, the record of safe usage and familiarity with prescribed medications that could interact with the herb in question. In contrast, academic institutions are obliged to regard each herb(s) as though it were a medication(s), with its own benefits and potential side effects that have to be weighed in general terms.

Placebo Effect(s)

The use of placebos has become standard practice as controls in clinical trials.[4,26,27,38,45,51] A recent position paper from the World Health Medical Association has advocated restrictions on the use of placebos based on ethical grounds.[21] This proposal has met with strong opposition from science, industry and federal regulators. Adding fuel to this debate is another paper that challenges whether there is even a placebo effect.[20,21] Unfortunately for this argument, the meta-analysis on which this conclusion is based can be faulted on several grounds, especially, the heterogeneity of the population on which the meta-analysis was based. In this case, the evidence to discount the existence of a placebo effect is not convincing.

More to the point seems to be the question of the role played by placebo effects in mediating the efficacy of complementary therapie[25,35] An associated question is how do placebos exert their effects?[5,13] The latter question was addressed at a recent conference sponsored by the National Institutes of Health.[1] At this meeting, investigators operating as part of the MacArthur Network summarized the results of a ten-year study concerned with mind-body-health interplay. Since the meeting, a new initiative has begun to explore the placebo effect using brain imaging, computer modeling and peripheral markers, such as neuroimmunological and neurohumoral mediators in blood. Even more recently, the National Institutes of Health have begun to issue RFAs designed to promote research on how placebos exert their mind-body-health effects.

Proper Usage

Few medical institutions either carry herbs in their pharmacies or have set standards for the practice of unconventional therapies. With respect to herbs, the situation is unlikely to change until federal legislation recognizes that herbs should be considered as medications rather than as foods.[18,29,30] At present, herbal products are readily available in food stores with no guarantee of uniformity of composition, concentration of effective ingredients, quality or freedom from contaminants.[54]

Other complementary therapies are less difficult than herbs to evaluate and control. Although licensing for hands-on therapies such as acupuncture can vary from state to state, guidelines concerning proper credentialing for practice are often available from specialty organizations, from consensus groups and from collections of evidence-based data, such as those in the Cochrane Collections.[19]

Qualified Personnel

As a rule medical schools are not densely populated with practitioners of complementary therapies. As a result, little opportunity is provided for exposure to the concepts and practices that derive from other cultures. Since there is no bustling academic pipeline of candidates for mentoring and training in complementary therapies, the void in experienced practitioners will have to be filled for a while mostly by practitioners of unconventional therapies drawn from the community.[8]

Academic medical institutions are currently responding to this need in two ways: 1) recruiting individual practitioners to teach and demonstrate complementary therapies and 2) affiliating with health professional schools that teach and practice unconventional therapies. Both of these recourses require that academic medical centers set standards for practice consistent with the guidelines and regulations that currently govern the practice of conventional medicine.

The Need for Research

As noted above, the need for research on complementary therapies is great but handicapped by lack of standardization of individual therapies and by a shortage of scientists trained to conduct research on unconventional therapies according to the principles and process of scientific medicine. Moreover, few practitioners of complementary therapies have been provided with incentives for systematic research.

Fortunately, this situation is improving both in response to popular demand and to incentives emanating from the National Center for Complementary/Alternative Medicine of the National Institutes of Health.

Conclusions

A pressing need exists for western medicine to assess complementary therapies for incorporation into conventional medical practice[32]. However, for this incorporation to occur, unconventional therapies will have to be tested, one-by-one, to satisfy western criteria for evidence-based medicine.[2,15,16,33] These criteria are embodied in long-standing western requirements for proof of safety, efficacy and, more recently, of cost-effectiveness.

Because scientific medicine and complementary medicine are currently not on equal footing, a stage of incorporation can be expected to precede the stage of integration. The process of incorporation followed by integration is occurring while western medicine is, *per se*, undergoing remarkable adaptive changes. Medical horizons have enlarged from acute to chronic illnesses, from preoccupation with cure to increasing concern about quality of life, and from heavy reliance on hospitals to practice and education in ambulatory settings.

All the above impacts on the education of the physician. The over-crowded curriculum has to make room for therapies currently regarded as unconventional and unproven but destined to become evidence-based as soon as proof of safety, efficacy and cost-effectiveness become available. Part of the process of integration will call for increased awareness of cultural diversity. And with the process of integration and increased awareness comes the prospect of heightened regard for the Hippocratic tradition and of increased professionalism in the practice of medicine.

References

1. Abbott, L.J., Ader, D.N. Ader, R. et al. The science of the placebo: toward and inter-disciplinary research agenda. NIH Center for CAM. Bethesda, MD. Nov. 19-21, 2000.

2. Angell, M., Kassirer, J.P. Alternative medicine - the risks of untested and unregulated remedies. *N Engl J Med*. 1998;339:839-41.

3. Astin, J.A. Why patients use alternative medicine: results of a national study. *JAMA*. 1998;279:1548-1553.

4. Beecher, H.K. The powerful placebo. *JAMA*. 1955;159:1602-1606.

5. Berns, G.S., et al. Predictability modulates human brain response to reward. *J. Neuroscience*, 2001;21:2793-2798.

6. Blendon, R.J., DesRoches, C.M., Benson, J.M. et al. Americans' views on the use and regulation of dietary supplements. *Arch Int Med*. 2001;161:805-810.

7. British Medical Association. <u>Complementary Medicine: New Approaches to Good Practice</u>. New York, Oxford University Press, 1993.

8. Cooper, R.A., Prakash, L., Dietrich, C.L., Current and projected workforce of non-physician clinicians. *JAMA* 1998;280:788-794.

9. Davidoff, F. Weighing the alternatives: lessons from the paradoxes of alternative medicine. *Ann Int Med*. 1998;129:1061-1065.

10. Eisenberg, D.M., Davis, R.B., Ettner, S.L., et al. Trends in alternative medicine use in the United States. 1990-1997:results of a follow-up national survey. *JAMA* 1998;280:1569-1574.

11. Eisenberg, D.M., Kessler, R.C., Foster, C., et al. Unconventional medicine in the Unites States. Prevalence, costs, and patterns of use. *N Engl J Med*. 1993;328:246-252.

12. Ernst, E. Harmless herbs? *Am J Med*. 1998;104:170-178.

13. Ernst, E., Barnes, J. Meta-analysis of homeopathy trials. *Lancet*. 1998;351:355-367.

14. Ezzo, J, Berman, B.M., Vickers, A.J., Linde, K. Complementary medicine and the Cochrane Collabo.ration. *JAMA*. 1998;280:1628-1630.

15. Federspil, G. and Vettor, R. Can Scientific Medicine - Incorporate Alternative Medicine? *J Alt Comp Med*. 2000;6:241-244.

16. Fontanarosa, P.B. and Lundberg, G.D. Alternative medicine meets science. *JAMA*. 1998;280:1618-1619.

17. Fuller, R.C. <u>Alternative Medicine and American Religious Life</u>. New York: Oxford University Press, 1995.

18. Goldman, P. Herbal medicines today and the roots of modern pharmacology. *Ann Int Med.* 2001;135:593-600.

19. Gordon, S. The regulation of complementary medicine. *Consumer Policy Review.* 1997;7:65-69.

20. Hrobjartsson, A. and Gotzsche, P.C. Is the placebo powerless? An analysis of clinical trials comparing placebo with no treatment. *N Eng J Med.* 2001;344:1594-1602.

21. Hust, P. and Peterson, R. Withholding proven treatment in clinical research. *N Eng J Med.* 2001;345:912-913.

22. *JAMA.* Special issue on Evaluating Alternative Therapies. 1998;18;11 November.

23. Jobst, K.A. Obstacles to healing in medicine and science: the interplay of science, paradigm and culture. *J Altern Complement Med.* 1999; 5:391-394.

24. Jonas, W.B. Alternative medicine - learning form the past, examining the present, advancing to the future. *JAMA.* 280:1616-1617.

25. Jonas, W.B. The homeopathy debate. Letter to the Editor, *J Alt Comp Med.* 2000;6:213-215.

26. Kaptchuk, T.J. Intentional ignorance: a history of blind assessment and placebo controls in medicine. *Bull Hist Med.* 1998;72;389-433.

27. Kaptchuk, T.J. The double-blind, randomized, placebo-controlled trial: gold standard or golden calf. *J Clin Endo.* 2001;54:541-549.

28. Kaptchuk, T.J., Eisenberg, D.M. The persuasive appeal of alternative medicine. *Ann Int Med.* 1998;129:1061-1065.

29. Kessler, D.A. Cancer and herbs. *N Engl J Med.* 2000;342:1742-1743.

30. Kessler, R.C., Davis, R.B., Foster, D.F., Van Rompay, M.I., Walters, E.E., Wilkey, S.A., et al. Long-term trends in the use of complementary and alternative medical therapies in the United States. *Ann Intern Med.* 2001;135:262-268.

31. Kienle, G.S. and Kiene, H. The powerful placebo: fact or fiction. *J Clin Epidem.* 1997;50:1311-1318.

32. Lawrence, L., Weisz, G. <u>Greater Than the Parts: Holism in Biomedicine</u> (1920-1950). New York: Oxford University Press, 1998.

33. Levin, J.S., Glass, T.A., Kushi, L.H. et al. Quantitative methods in research oncomplementary and alternative medicine. *Med Care.* 1997;35:1079-1094.

34. Lewith, G. and Aldridge. Complementary Medicine and the European Community. Saffron Walden: C.W. Daniel Co., 1991, pp 45-60.

35. Linde, K, Clausius, N, Ramirez, G., et al. Are the clinical effects of homeopathy trials placebo effects? A meta-analysis of homeopathy trials. *Lancet.* 1998;351:366-367.

36. MacPherson, H. Fatal and adverse events from acupuncture: allegation, evidence and the implications. *J Altern Complement Med.* 1991;5:223-224.

37. Marcus, D.M. How should alternative medicine be taught to medical students and physicians? *Acad Med.* 2001;76:224-229.

38. Mattocks, K.M, Horwitz, RI. Placebos, active control groups, and the unpredictability paradox. *Biol. Psychiatry.* 2000;47:693-698.

39. Medical School Objectives Project. Report I: Learning Objectives for Medical Student Education-Guidelines for Medical Schools. Washington, DC: Association of American Medical Colleges, 1998.

40. Milan, F.B., Landau, C., Murphy, D.R., et al. Teaching residents about complementary and alternative medicine in the United States. *J Gen Intern Med.* 1999; 13:562-567.

41. Moerman, D.E. Cultural variations in the placebo effect: ulcers, anxiety and blood pressure. *Med Anthropology Quart.* 2000;14:51-72.

42. Nahin, R.I. and Straus, S.E. Research into complementary and alternative medicine: problems and potential. *BMJ.* 2001;7279:161-163.

43. Nortier, J.L., Martinez, MCM, Schmeiser, HH et al. Urothelial carcinoma associated with the use of a Chinese herb. *N Eng J Med.* 2000;342:1686-1692.

44. Ramsey, M. Alternative medicine in modern France. *Med-Hist.* 1999;43:286-322.

45. Reilly, D. Taylor, M.A., Beattie, N.G.M. et al. Is evidence for homeopathy reproducible? *The Lancet.* 1994; 344:1601-1606.

46. Popper, K.R. The Logic of Scientific Discovery. London: Hutchinson and Co., 1959.

47. Sackett, D.L., Rosenberg, W.M., Gray, J.A., et al. Evidence-based medicine: what it is and what it isn't. *BMJ.* 1996;312:71-72.

48. Saks, M. Alternative Medicine in Britain. Oxford: Clarendon Press, 1991.

49. Sampson, W. The need for educational reform in teaching about alternative therapies. *Acad Med.* 2001;76:248-250.

50. Shelton, R.C., Keller, M.B., Gelenberg, A. et al. Effectiveness of St. John's Wort in major depression. *JAMA* 2001;285:1978-1985

51. Temple, R., Ellenberg, S.S. Placebo-controlled trials and active-controlled trials in the evaluation of new treatments. *Ann Int Med.* 2000;133:455-463.

52. Tulder, M.W., van, Cherkin, D.C., Berman, B. et al. Acupuncture for low back pain. *The Cochrane Collaboration.* 1999.

53. Vickers, A. Evidence-based medicine and complementary medicine. *ACP Journal Club.* 1999;130:A-13-14.

54. Vogel, G. How the body's "garbage disposal" may inactivate drugs. *Science.* 2001;291:35-37.

55. Wetzel, M.S., Eisenberg, D.M., Kaptchuk, T.J. Courses involving complementary and alternative medicine at US medical schools. *JAMA.* 1998;280:784-787.

56. Wilt, T.J., Ishani, A., Stark, G. et al. Saw palmetto extracts for treatment of benign prostatic hyperplasia: a systematic review. *JAMA.* 1998; 280:1604-1609.

57. Young, J.H. The development of the Office of Alternative Medicine in the National Institutes of Health 1991-1996. *Bull Hist Med.* 1998;72:279-298.

Why Is There a Conflict Between Complementary/Alternative Medicine and the Medical Establishment?

Leon Eisenberg, M.D.
Harvard Medical School

Preface

The reasons for the conflict between complementary/alternative medicine (CAM) and the medical establishment (ME) are geopolitical (turf, money, and prestige) and epistemological (the nature of evidence and the disconfirmability of theory). Before I examine those issues in some detail, prefatory comments are appropriate.

First of all, CAM and ME are not uniform camps unified against an external enemy. To lump all CAM practitioners together is a classificatory fiction like the category, "Hispanic," in the census; it lumps together Cubans and Puerto Ricans simply because both speak Spanish (or, worse, because their parents spoke Spanish!). They differ from each other by education, social class, and health status by more than "Hispanics" do from "Caucasians." In like fashion, herbalists, chiropractors, spiritists, exorcists and acupuncturists are grouped as "irregular" or "unconventional" practitioners; they differ from each other as much as they differ from physicians.[1] Licensed practitioners make up a more homogeneous category (80 percent are graduates of accredited US medical schools), but lumping glosses over important differences between academics and practitioners, specialists and generalists, those in salaried and those in fee-for-service practice. In the discussion that follows, I will, for the most part, ignore the subdivisions within the warring camps.

Secondly, whatever the balance between CAM and ME in the market place, the therapeutic power of biomedicine far outweighs that of alternative healing practices for most life-threatening diseases. The younger members of this audience cannot appreciate the changes in medicine during the past century. At its beginning, infectious diseases were the leading cause of death. Until the 1930's, doctors had been impotent in the face of bacterial infection; chemotherapy and antibiotics revolutionized care. So rapid was the change that Surgeon General Stewart told Congress in 1969 that it was time to "close the book on infectious disease." Stewart was wrong, very wrong, but the quote indicates the euphoria aroused by progress (Cohen 2000). When I graduated from medical school, the diagnosis of acute lymphocytic leukemia in children was tantamount to a death warrant; only 10 percent were alive two years later. Now survival at five years is 80 percent. Age-specific death rates from cardiovascular disease and stroke have been markedly reduced, in part because of biomedical interventions, in part because of effective prevention through public health programs. Consider the greater quality of life total hip replacement brings to patients with painful and immobilizing osteoarthritis. There are many hundreds of such examples. The point is that these beneficial changes stem from science applied to patient care (Eisenberg 1997). Rigorous science has been notably absent from complementary/alternative medicine.

Why has dissatisfaction with American medicine become so vociferous at the very time doctors control powerful medical technology? The "old-fashioned general practitioner," with few drugs that worked and not much surgery that did, looks good to many patients (in retrospect, of course).[II] How can we explain the paradox that more effective medicine has resulted in lay nostalgia for a medically impotent past?

Medicine has too narrow a view of what is "scientific," an unwarranted belief in "specificity" and a disdain for the interpersonal aspects of medical care. The very virtuosity of the new technology has resulted in a focus on machines instead of patients. Diseases that are chronic, recurrent, and defy cure are the ones for which physicians do the worst and alternative practitioners the best. Joel Dimsdale (1999), the editor of *Psychosomatic Medicine* has suggested that "in many ways, alternative medicine is the mirror image of traditional medicine – strong on caring and weak on science."

Outline

With no pretense at being neutral but with due regard for the evidence,[III] I have organized this presentation around nine issues: satisfying patients; harming patients; geopolitics; epistemologic differences; science in theory and practice (the culture of science); treating disease and treating illness; the randomized controlled trial as the gold standard; the difference between efficacy and effectiveness; and can the war be won?

Satisfying Patients

> The secret of the care of the patient is in caring for the patient.
> —Francis W. Peabody (1930)

Most patients recover from most illness episodes most of the time. Most chronic illnesses undergo periodic remissions and exacerbations at unpredictable times; a remission following an intervention is attributed by patients and doctors to the treatment. For millennia, those happy facts have enabled folk healers and doctors to receive credit from their patients for recovery during their ministrations. This characteristic of healing practices was recognized in Imperial China more than 2000 years ago bt the Chief Physician of the Imperial Government:

> the I Shih, in charge of the whole medical administration of the country,...uses the records of each physician to decide on his rank and salary. Those who have cured 100 percent of their patients are graded in the first class, those who have 90 percent recoveries are placed in the second class, those 80 percent successful are placed third, those who cured 70 percent are considered fourth class, and the lowest grade of all contains those who could not cure more than 60 percent.

A later commentator on the text explained the rating system:

> The reason why those who failed with four out of ten patients were placed in the lowest grade was because half the cases might well have recovered anyway even without any treatment at all (Needham 1981).

The patient whose symptoms remit is ready to credit the doctor; the doctor is happy to accept it. But spontaneous remission is not the whole story. Relief may follow from the very act of consultation because of belief in the doctor's therapeutic virtuosity. Relief follows from being cared for (Peabody 1930), from having one's worst fears dismissed, from being given a treatment program (something to do to make matters better) all part of what is dismissed as "clinical management." The process is self-reinforcing. Each experience of benefit enhances the likelihood of subsequent benefit. Paradoxically, the very accomplishments produced by scientific research have augmented medicine's power as metaphor and magic. Medical theories are incorporated in the general culture. As has ever been true, explanation diminishes the discomfort from illness, whether those explanations are speculative or data based. Patients come to the healer seeking meaning to diminish perplexity in the face of distress. When the doctor pronounces that the fever is due to a "virus," both patient and doctor find the "diagnosis" comforting even in the complete absence of virological studies (Eisenberg 1987). The disorder has a name; it fits into a frame of meaning; it is no longer evil or malignant. In non-Western cultures, the naming of other "diagnoses" (syntonic with each culture) plays the same role when the syndrome is attributed to taboo violation, an offense against an ancestor, witchcraft, spirit possessions or other such supernatural phenomena.

Biomedicine summarily dismisses "nonspecific" treatment effects (effects not attributable to the known pharmacological action of a drug) to "placebo," a Latin verb meaning "I please." *Dorland's Medical Dictionary* defines placebo as "an inactive substance given to satisfy the patient's symbolic need for drug therapy..., a procedure with no intrinsic therapeutic value." That definition dismisses utterly the value of the care and caring provided by the healers who provide the treatment. In a clinical trial, the placebo is used to control for (a) secular changes in illness course and (b) improvement resulting from care. To attribute:

> clinical improvement solely to placebo effects...is an insult to the importance of caring. It diverts attention from the fundamental need always to provide optimum caring as a necessary basis for technical intervention... Compliant participation in any controlled trial, whether in its placebo, or actively treated, wing almost invariably improves outcome even if measured by mortality... The effects of downgrading and neglect of caring by research theory have been magnified by market incentives... Caring has been central to medical practice in all cultures throughout history... (Hart and Dieppe 1996)

This was powerfully demonstrated, entirely by inadvertence, in a clinical trial of clofibrate, a drug introduced to diminish risk factors for coronary heart disease (Coronary Project Group 1980). Among the thousand men who received the drug, those who took their pills as directed showed a substantially lower five-year mortality than did those who failed to do so (15 percent vs. 25 percent). Had the analysis ended there, clofibrate would have been hailed as a wonder drug. However, the double-blind study design included 2700 men given a lactose placebo. Among those who took their placebo as directed, the mortality was 15 percent (vs. 29 percent among non-compliers). Clofibrate was unrelated to the outcome. Patients who followed the doctor's orders had a significantly different lower mortality from those who did not. Why? Did treatment adherence merely serve as a marker for otherwise undetected biological characteristics related to mortality? Or did the mortality difference reflect changes in habits (in smoking, diet, exercise, and the like), more probable among compliant patients enrolled in a heart disease trial? The question can not be answered; the necessary information was not collected. To the investigators, the placebo was a "control." They measured compliance only to be sure the experimentals were taking their clofibrate. The trial was a disappointment to the pharmacologists; the drug didn't work. But it should have been a cause for celebration: they had shown that a behavioral characteristic produced benefits far in excess of those expectable from excellent medications!

Harming Patients

Is the difference between CAM and ME a matter of ethics? Great acrimony is aroused in both camps by accusations of unethical behavior. The fact that some CAM practitioners are dishonest, unscrupulous and dangerous no more settles the case than the fact that some medical practitioners exhibit the same traits. Unscrupulous providers prey upon patients with ill-defined and chronic disorders. On which side of the fence are more quacks to be found? I am not aware of any empirical evidence on the matter. CAM practitioners who fleece their clients make the news I read more often, but physicians do so poor a job of policing colleagues that reliable information on the extent of medical malfeasance and malpractice is not to be found (Editorial 2000).

Charlatans with an M.D. Degree

The Wall Street Journal (Burton 1999) described neurosurgeons who are drilling and removing bone from the occiput and adjacent spinal column to "decompress" the brain in patients with fibromyalgia and chronic fatigue syndrome. There is no evidence for "increased pressure" nor are there clinical data on the effectiveness of this invasive procedure. It is, however, lucrative (30,000 dollars per case). Reputable practitioners condemn it, but the doctors who do it continue to have hospital privileges.

Academic fraud of a more dangerous type was recently uncovered. Werner Bezwoda of the University of Witwatersand reported unusual success in two studies of patients with breast cancer placed on high-dose chemotherapy with autologous progenitor-cell transplantation. The finding encouraged replication because other randomized trials failed to show benefit. Before embarking on a trial involving thousands of women, a US team was deputized to make an on-site review (Weiss et al. 2000). The team found gross disparities between the information in patient records and the data Bezwoda presented at international meetings. Neither informed consent nor institutional approval had been obtained. Confronted with the evidence, Bezwoda acknowledged "scientific misconduct." What a pale description of a fraud that put lives at risk! The scientific community relies on trust and on replication. Research that claims to be a "breakthrough" is rapidly put to the test. Is trust misplaced?

The German Research Council (DFG) has investigated 347 papers published by a hematologist accused of fraud. The DFG task force concluded that ninety-four were definitely falsified, 121 may have been faked, and only 132 were "clean". The chairman of the hematology department was co-author on 59 of the papers; he said he was an "honorary author," unaware of experimental details. The investigative task force blamed lax German standards for clinical research and an academic environment that requires multiple publications before clinicians can be promoted (Abbott 2000).

If those tales exemplify unethical behavior by physicians, to whom do we assign blame for the cures promised by Dr. Luigi DiBella, a physician in Modena, Italy? DiBella promoted his multi-therapy (MDB) as a cancer cure. When the Ministry of Health refused to approve reimbursement for this unproven "treatment," (the ingredients were secret and there were no published data), a nationwide newspaper campaign accused the government of indifference to suffering. The resulting political upheaval forced the government to fund the fraudulent treatment. A clinical trial, undertaken with DiBella's reluctant participation, showed no benefit; he disputed the findings on the grounds that his protocol had not been followed "precisely." When the Ministry undertook a systematic follow up of the patients treated by DiBella during the previous 25 years, five-year survival proved to be <u>lower</u> in patients who received MDB as a supplement to standard treatment (Buiatti et al. 1999). DiBella is an MD who capitalized on an ineffectual and hazardous nostrum sold to desperate patients as an "alternative treatment." The Italian medical establishment opposed DiBella. To which camp shall we apportion this fraud?

CAM Quacks

There is no way to document the harm to patients resulting from delay in seeking medical treatment when the patient's initial and/or continuing resort is to CAM. For diseases with optimal medical therapy, the use of CAM as an alternative to medical treatment is clearly detrimental to patient health. Some healers do refer inappropriate cases; many don't; some don't recognize what they are seeing; others believe they can work miracles; still others are simply venal. How many fall into each category? Facts are lacking.

CAM enthusiasts perpetuate the myth that herbs and dietary supplements are safer than conventional medicines because they are "organic" or "natural" and contain no man-made chemicals. Perversely, the belief in safety and lack of side effects is abetted by physicians who dismiss natural products as inert and useless. Some have active ingredients; some are highly toxic. Yellow oleander is a plant common in the tropics and subtropics. Ingestion of sufficient quantities leads to digoxin poisoning. Deliberate self-poisoning with yellow oleander has become a major public health problem in Sri Lanka (Eddleston et al 2000).

The Chinese herb *Aristolochia fangchi* has been implicated in an epidemic of rapidly progressing interstitial nephritis and urothelial cancer in Belgian patients using herbal slimming pills (Nortier et al. 2000). The nephrotoxic substance in the herb is aristolochic acid, which is a carcinogen. Among 39 patients with kidney failure after taking the herbal pills, 18 had evidence of cancer, and 19 of the remaining 21 had signs of tissue damage. Other well-documented examples of severe adverse reactions include the association of germander with acute hepatitis, of comfrey with hepatic veno-occlusive disease, of yohimbe with seizures and renal failure, and of ephedra with death from cardiovasular disease (Kessler 2000).

The 1994 Dietary Supplement Act (passed after heavy lobbying by the industry) classifies "botanicals" as food supplements and does not require that they be shown to be safe or effective before they are marketed. The FDA can only act after the fact (Kessler 2000). Even straightforward trials of "botanicals" face severe hurdles. There is no assurance of the quality and consistency of the product being tested; the active ingredient may not be known, let alone its bioavailability or shelf-life.

Fugh-Berman (2000) has reviewed the evidence on herb-drug inter-actions. Concurrent use of herbs may mimic, magnify or oppose drug effects. Over-the-counter preparations vary in purity, in the amount of active substance they contain, and in cost (McAlindon et al. *JAMA* 2000; 283:1469-75). Mixing herbs and prescription drugs can be dangerous to your health.

Who is at greatest risk from CAM practices? In August 2000, the Queens District Attorney shut down the "New York Beijing Hospital of Traditional Chinese Medicine" for operating without a license and without licensed physicians (though it advertised having them). The authorities learned of it after a patient, infected by a gynecologic procedure, sued for malpractice and was told, "the doctors couldn't be sued because they didn't have licenses!" The "doctors" wore white coats, carried stethoscopes and tended to patients on examin-ing tables, the paraphernalia of medicine. They prescribed herbs and Chinese food supplements. (Kershaw 2000). Who did they vic-timize? Poor undocumented aliens, people just like them. Cultural congruence is no guarantee of adequate care.

Thousands of similar clinics patronized by immigrants flourish in New York City. "Stymied by a lack of health insurance, fearful (of being reported to immigration authorities), and longing for familiar remedies dispensed by someone who speaks their language, many of the city's immigrants have been driven to create their own complex methods of getting health care" (Steinhauer 2000). The practitioners include herbal healers, voodoo priests, pharmacists who double as doctors, shamans who perform exorcisms, purveyors of magic amulets and suppliers of illegally obtained and unwisely used antibiotics. Forty percent of *legal* immigrants are uninsured; the percentage is far higher among undocumented aliens. For many, CAM is not a matter of preference but the consequence of barriers to conventional medicine.

Does Good Faith Guarantee Good Outcomes?

There are, in both camps, conscientious practitioners who follow the precepts of their trade in good faith and those who either don't know or don't care whether the client is helped or harmed, so long as they are paid. Sincerity, however, does not ensure beneficence.

The American physician Benjamin Rush, the first Surgeon General of the United States, threw himself into the breech during an epidemic of yellow fever in Philadelphia in 1793. Panic beset the city; more than a third of its population of 50,000 fled to the surrounding countryside; before the plague receded, more than 4,000 lives were lost. Many doctors fled. Of those who remained, ten died of the disease. From illness and defection, only three physicians were available to treat some 6,000 patients!

Rush, after dispatching his wife and children to a safe area, stayed behind to fulfill his medical obligations. Believing that yellow fever resulted from an "excitement of the blood," he ministered to his patients by vigorous bleeding and purging. Desperate diseases required desperate remedies. In the midst of his rounds, he fell ill with the fever. He had his assistant apply his remedy to himself. He was bled several times leaving him "in so weak a state, I woke two successive nights with a faintness which threatened the extinction of my life.....my convalescence was extremely slow." His recovery affirmed his conviction that his methods were right. Inspired by the best of motives, Rush probably hastened the demise of many of his patients (Middleton 1928).

Blood letting treatment persisted well into the 19th century. It was not discarded until the French physician Pierre Louis introduced the "numerical method" (that is, statistics) into medicine (Eisenberg 1997). His precise observations, his collection of case series, and his insistence on testing received wisdom influenced medical practice. American physicians who went to Paris for study returned to these shores convinced of the utility of the numerical method. If Rush and the yellow fever caution us that meaning well is not the same thing as doing well, Louis and the numerical method remind us that scientific medicine has, when it uses it, a method to separate clinical truth from fiction.

The romantic view of folk healers depicts a community bound by long tradition that uses the wisdom possessed by shamans to cure illnesses. However, the belief system of many pre-literate peoples holds that shamans and witch doctors can cast spells able to cause disease as well as cure it. The management of sickness episodes can become a way of dramatizing and resolving mounting social tensions within the community by using the accusations of witchcraft to destroy the legitimacy of one of the competing factions (Young 1976). Given the imprecision of folk illness categories, the sick person and his family can seek diagnosticians of different "specialties." Turner

(1975) concluded from his studies of Ndembu healers in rural Zambia that:

> from the Ndembu point of view…the diviner is a man who redresses breaches in the social order, enunciates moral law, detects those who secretly and malevolently transgress it, and prescribes remedial action…

> Healers, living in the community and acutely aware of the tensions and enmities within it, do not plant accusations randomly but rather know, before divination ceremonies begin, the enemies and the allies of the patient's family.

The belief in sorcery as a major cause of illness wreaks havoc during a disease epidemic which cannot be "controlled" by magic. Lindenbaum (1979) has described the crisis provoked by the spread of kuru among the Southern Fore in the Eastern Highlands of Papua New Guinea. Kuru is an invariably fatal progressive disease of the central nervous system caused by (in the western meaning of cause) a prion, an infectious proteinaceous particle. In the medical classification scheme of the Fore, kuru is one of a group of diseases caused by the malicious actions of human sorcerers. Accordingly, the appropriate response to a case of kuru in the family is to summon a curer to identify the sorcerer and offset his malignant influences by appropriate magical remedies. As the pandemic intensified, accusations and suspicions mounted: curers themselves were denounced as frauds because their rituals failed to heal; villagers turned against one another; warfare was imminent. Unable to control the disease at the local level, the Fore assembled in mass meetings known as kibungs. The sorcerers were publicly reproached for crimes against society and urged to confess their misdeeds; some public "confessions" were indeed elicited (a phenomenon like the confessions elicited in totalitarian states). Speakers called for brotherhood and unity:

> Our ancestors were the same. We living men are the ones
> who split apart and gave separate names to our groups.
> At this kibung let us adopt the customs of our ancestors.
> We will stop making kuru on our own people. Ibubuli is
> our all inclusive name (Lindenbaum, ibid)

The kibungs served to minimize internecine warfare but they, too, fell into disuse as disease persisted. It took modern laboratory techniques to identify a potential agent and a mode of transmission

When modernization and legal regulation gradually transformed the social customs of the Fore, kuru was controlled; transmission was interrupted by ending the practice of ritual cannibalism as a rite of mourning and respect for dead kinsmen.

Geopolitics

> War is nothing more than the continuation of politics by
> other means.   —Karl Von Clausewitz: On War (1832)

I now turn to the geopolitical (turf, money and prestige) factors in the "war" between ME and CAM. Asked why there is a war, physicians might begin by objecting to the metaphor of "war" and substitute "police action". As they see it, they are engaged in protecting a gullible and scientifically illiterate public from snake oil salesmen and quacks. They point to the absence of credible scientific evidence on the effectiveness of CAM. They dismiss CAM "theories" as patently absurd because they violate established scientific principles. Acupuncture is a case in point. The meridians supposed to indicate loci for needle insertion do not correspond with the facts of Vesalian anatomy and are just as fanciful as were phrenological maps of brain function derived from palpating bumps on the skull. [This dismissal of the theory of acupuncture is, however, quite different from whether, and under what circumstances, acupuncture works and, if it does, why.] Were the same question put to CAM practitioners, they would highlight the economic self interest of physicians out to protect their turf. As far as CAM is concerned, scientific "principles" are irrelevant. They <u>know</u> from experience that their treatments work. As to contradicting "Science," they insist that there are more things in heaven and earth than are dreamt of in medical philosophy.

Turf, Money, And Prestige

Why should the medical establishment, so powerful and wealthy, fight so bitterly against fringe practitioners whose assets are so limited trial lawyers usually do not bother to sue them? That antagonism is rooted in history. For most of the nineteenth century, there were no licensure laws in the US. American society was anti-elitist; states refused to grant exclusive privileges to one group. The result was "market place professionalism," at quite a remove from older European models (Mohr 2000). Each healer had to shift for him/herself as did each patient. Physicians hustled for business in a market that included a spectrum of alternative and antagonistic healers, some trained and others simply self-proclaimed.

There were medical schools of many persuasions and uncertain quality producing far too many practitioners. The American Medical Association fought to upgrade the level of medical education (and to reduce competition in the medical marketplace) by closing marginal proprietary schools, a move accelerated by the 1910 Flexner Report. In the following decade, one third of medical schools closed. Between 1900 and 1920, the number of graduates fell by half and did not reach the 1900 total again until 1950. The AMA fought relentlessly against increasing class size and opening new schools. Its leadership had been scarred by the depression of the 1930s when many family doctors barely made a living (Richmond 1969).

Not until the 1920s did all states have medical licensure laws limiting practice to graduates of approved medical schools. In the '30s and '40s, the profession consolidated control of practice in advance of substantial therapeutic gains. Paul Beeson (1980) compared the treatments recommended in the first (1927) edition of *Cecil's Textbook of Medicine* with those in its 14th (1975) edition. By 1980 standards, Beeson rated the value of <u>60 percent</u> of the remedies in the first edition as harmful, dubious, or merely symptomatic; only 3 percent provided fully effective treatment or prevention. In the 48-year interval between the two editions, effective regimens had increased seven-fold and the dubious ones had decreased by two-thirds. Post-war advances in chemotherapy, surgery, and diagnostic methods made doctors (relatively speaking) miracle workers; palpable gains in efficacy made ME dominant.

Yet, complementary and alternative medicine continues to control a large and growing consumer market. In 1997, 42 percent of Americans had tried some sort of alternative medicine, an increase from the 34 percent recorded in 1990. In 1997, Americans spent 27 billion dollars on unproven remedies (Eisenberg et al. 1998). In that year, total national health expenditures exceeded a trillion dollars; of that amount, 20 percent was reimbursement for physician services (National Center for Health Statistics 1998). The amounts spent on CAM can be computed as 3 percent of total costs, and seem small – or as 13 percent of physician costs, and seem large. Senator Dirksen of Illinois famously said on the Senate floor: "You spend a billion here and a billion there and before you know it, it adds up to real money." Physicians agree: CAM costs are adding up to real money.

But is the frequency of use of CAM as high as 42 percent? Druss and Rosenheck (1999) estimated use at 8.3 percent. They found that most CAM users also visit physicians; moreover, high utilizers of conventional care were much more likely to turn to CAM as well.[IV] Ernst (2000), after reviewing the prevalences reported in international journals, identified "rates" varying from 9 percent to 65 percent. Soberly, he concluded that frequency of use remains to be determined.

Are There Possibilities for a Negotiated Settlement?

Are there possibilities for a truce and a negotiated settlement in this war? Early signs suggest a new amity. Medical schools are establishing Departments or Divisions of CAM. Elective CAM courses are offered by two-thirds of American medical schools (Wetzel et al. 1999). Another harbinger of the new Spring is the appointment of Stephen Straus, M.D., a senior NIH investigator, to direct the National Center for Complementary and Alternative Medicine (NCCAM) for the scientific study of widely used remedies to (Stokstad 2000). NCCAM has to satisfy CAM believers like Senator Harkin of Iowa and Representative Burton of Indiana, who upped its funding, and academics like Wallace Sampson of Stanford, who dismiss NCCAM "as an employment agency for opportunists and a source for aberrant and biased science." It remains to be seen whether the Center and its Director can survive if the studies NCCAM funds alienate the CAM constituency that gave it birth.

Hospitals and clinics across the country are beginning to provide CAM services on the premises. This is not an "evidence driven" decision but a maneuver to increase market leverage akin to providing hospital amenities. *The New York Times* (La Perla 2000) describes the reception room of the Rockefeller Pavilion at the Memorial Sloan-Kettering Cancer Center as "part luxury hotel, part Zen-like retreat." It is, she writes, the "aesthetic equivalent of acupuncture." Some health care institutions now offer on-site hair salons, Zen tea rooms, mellow lighting, waterfalls, vanilla-scented candles, and seagrass. The outpatient clinic of the Beth Israel Medical Center in New York offers medical care alongside Eastern therapies in an environment described as "Hong Kong hotel style." A group of privately practicing dermatologists with teaching hospital affiliations recently announced opening a "vein and laser center" for removal of unattractive hair, facial and leg veins and red spots, adding that "our senior aesthetician [offers] chemical peels, microdermabrasion, make-up applications, facials and consultations regarding skin care [including] several lines of skin care products that we offer." It is not that "the morality of cosmetic surgery for aging" (Ringel 1998) has gone unchallenged but that the challenge has been unavailing. Dr. Ringel points out that cosmetic procedures have become an integral part of dermatologic practice whereas that was quite uncommon twenty years ago. Because cosmetic procedures are invasive, potentially morbid techniques with implications that go far beyond their commercial value as "practice builders," Dr. Ringel calls upon her fellow dermatologists "to explore the moral and psychosocial as well as the scientific and technical implications of the procedures they perform."

Whether the claim in the Times article that "patients who look at boats and beaches in pre-op do much better in surgery" is true or not, all of us prefer pleasant surroundings. What is driving the inclusion of amenities is not new data but competition for patients in the marketplace. That force, far more than an appreciation of the therapeutic value of CAM, drives hospitals to offer it. When a neuro-surgical service at a university hospital provides "therapeutic touch" as part of its "package" of patient care, this is not evidence-driven [such evidence as there is, is negative], but bottom-line driven. This sudden conversion undercuts the ME claim that its opposition to CAM has been based on science rather than economics. Many academic physicians are dismayed at this accommodation to the demands of the market, but the control of the academic medical center has passed from the faculty to medical administrators (Eisenberg 1999).

Epistemology

> One of the chief causes of poverty in science is imaginary wealth. The purpose of science is not to open the door to an infinitude of wisdom, but to set some limits on the infinitude of error. —Bertholt Brecht, *Life of Galileo.*

All theories of disease are attempts to order the puzzling phenomena of illness by invoking the hidden workings of invisible first principles, whether those principles be: spirit possession, yin and yang, viruses, or mutated genes. As Robin Horton (1967) has pointed out: "The quest for explanatory theory is basically the quest for unity underlying apparent diversity; for simplicity underlying apparent complexity; for order underlying apparent disorder; for regularity underlying apparent anomaly." All medical theories, traditional as well as Western, invoke invisible first principles, but the systems differ in their response when challenged. The elements of traditional beliefs are imbedded in fundamental dogma; they cannot be discarded without discarding the entire belief system much like the belief in Biblical inerrancy among some fundamentalist Baptists. The Bible says that the Lord created the earth and the creatures on it in six days and rested on the seventh. If that is taken as literal truth rather than metaphor, astrophysics, geology, and evolutionary biology must be false, whatever practical results they yield. The Pope may have remitted Galileo's conviction for heresy four centuries after the event, but the Kansas Board of Education banned the teaching of evolution just last year.

CAM theories rest on tradition, "This is the way our ancestors did it;" authority, "This is what my teacher told me;" and experience, "I have seen it work." Where written texts exist, as in Ayurveda or homeopathy, they are the final authority. Most CAM traditions are transmitted orally. One can acknowledge that folk wisdom does represent cumulative knowledge, but it includes unwinnowed chaff. The common-sense belief, shared by many pre-literate cultures the world over, that diarrhea should be treated by restricting oral intake can be fatal for infants and children. No remedy has been more effective than the UNICEF oral rehydration treatment that defies "common sense" and saves lives.

Faith-based and science-based systems are incommensurable in theory and practice. Consider Christian Science assertion that faith can cure disease. By definition, failure to respond results from insufficient faith. Thus, there is no way to challenge the circular proposition because there is no measure of "faith" independent of recovery. Distraught parents brought a malpractice suit against the Christian Science Church and two of its healing "practitioners" after their child died of bacterial meningitis. The practitioners had object-ed to medical consultation. Testifying on behalf of the Church, J. Thomas Black, current President of the Christian Science Church in Boston and First Reader in the Mother Church (Balliett 2000), stated that:

> Whenever Christian Science is *properly applied*, it
> heals...The parents...were much more intent on physical

healing than in spiritual growth and moral regeneration. [Christian Science] was therefore misapplied.

Believers in faith healing, spiritism, herbalism, Chinese medicine, and so on regard the canons of science as irrelevant. The scientist who disputes their claims has no way to put them to a decisive test. One can not "randomly assign" patients to faith healing vs. control conditions, not only because the treatments cannot be blinded, but because non-believers are hardly appropriate test subjects for faith healing. When treatment fails for believers, it is not the treatment that has failed, but the patient.

Precise diagnosis and description of the intervention are essential to the evaluation process. In alternative medicine, the mix of ingredients may vary in an unknown fashion between one herbal preparation and another. Similar caveats apply in cases where the charisma of the healer is an important ingredient in the treatment. CAM diagnosis may be based on systems incompatible with allopathic classification schemes. "Paralysis" can be cured by faith healing if the paralysis is caused by conversion hysteria; documentation of a cure in patients with transverse myelitis or spinal cord tumor is rare or absent.

Science in Theory and in Practice (The Culture of Science)

Science is a way of knowing, not a collection of facts. Science includes methods to disconfirm and discard specific hypotheses. A theory is scientific in so far as it is potentially disconfirmable; that is, it leads to predictions of events and findings that can be checked against expectation. International attention was focused on the 1913 eclipse of the sun because the phenomena to be observed would provide a critical test of Einstein's General Theory of Relativity, which predicted gravity would bend light, a counterintuitive supposition, one theretofore untestable. When astronomers reported that rays of light from distant stars were deflected by the sun's gravitational field, just as General Relativity required, the President of the Royal Society hailed the theory as "one of the greatest achievements in the history of human thought." (Frank 1947).

At least, that's the way the story is usually told. It is possible that the British astrophysicist, Sir Arthur Eddington, who was a champion of Einstein's theory, and who made the crucial observations of the solar eclipse, may have discarded some observations that didn't quite fit, believing them to be erroneous. It was not, mind you, that

Eddington fudged. Every experimentalist has to be sure his equipment is working properly; sometimes, "results" obviously represent equipment failure. But between "obviously" and "probably" and "possibly," exquisite judgment is required in making the distinctions. Eddington came down on the right side; subsequent studies all agree.

Physics is taken as the prototype of scientific objectivity and precision. But is it that cut and dried? Robert Millikan, the Chicago physicist who won a Nobel Prize for his work on the charge on the electron, was convinced before he began his experiments that the electron had a discrete charge (that is, that every electron had the same charge as every other one). Other reputable physicists were equally sure that the charge varied on a continuum among electrons; the obtained experimental values were thought to represent an average. Millikan's model guided his decisions about which experimental runs were "valid" and which were in "error." He published 58 experimental runs which were remarkably invariant, producing a value for the charge on the electron almost identical with the one in use today. However, his carefully preserved lab notebooks recorded 82 other experiments he didn't publish. His mental model guided his decisions about which findings were valid. Millikan was not, I repeat, cheating; if he had been a cheat, he would have destroyed his notebooks. His next project on the photoelectric effect began with incorrect presuppositions; he worked ten long years before abandoning it.

What about today? Experimental particle physicists are searching for events so rare that expectation has become as much a problem for them as it is for physicians in doing drug clinical trials. To reduce bias, research teams have had colleagues program their computers to add unknown numbers called "offsets" to their data to make their data analyses "blind." Only after the experiment is over do they discover what the "offset number" is to determine whether they have merely confirmed the obvious or have evidence for the elusive particle.

It is an injustice to science and scientists to fail to acknowledge the role of creative imagination at the frontiers of science. Two contemporaneous 17th century scientists, Harriot in London and Galileo in Padua, independently studied the moon with the telescope, a new invention from the Netherlands (Holton 1996). Since antiquity, the moon had been regarded as a perfectly smooth sphere, a symbol of an incorruptible universe. Harriot's drawings make it clear that he observed a jagged line at the division between the dark and illuminated portions of the moon, a line that should have been a smooth curve if the moon was perfect. He saw the "defect" and recorded it, but made no comment. Galileo saw similar irregularities on repeated observation as well as the numerous small bright areas within the dark part of the moon and dark areas in the bright part. Those observations led him to the remarkably bold conclusion that the blemishes represented prominences and cavities, like the mountains and valleys of the earth. From the shadows cast by the peaks, he calculated that some mountains on the moon were higher than the Alps. As Galileo's sensational findings spread through Europe, they transformed what other scientists "saw". Harriot himself, after reading Galileo, was able to see a mountainous moon.

Although scientists know that theories are provisional, in practice they come to mistake them for absolute. Scientific concepts are inventions of the imagination, not facts of nature. Adam Smith, the economist, wrote a treatise on the *History of Astronomy* (1790), which led him to conclude that:

> Philosophy is the science of the connecting principles of nature… Philosophy, by representing the invisible chains which bind together… disjointed objects, endeavors to introduce order into this chaos of jarring and discordant appearances, to allay this tumult of the imagination, and to restore it, when it surveys the great revolutions of the universe, to that tone of tranquility and composure, which is both most agreeable in itself and most suitable to its nature….

As he reviewed the successive astronomical theories from the Greeks to Newton, he recognized that each new account of the "invisible chains" provided a more coherent explanation than its predecessor; nevertheless, each was succeeded by an even more comprehensive act of the imagination.

Smith concluded:

> The system of Sir Isaac Newton is one whose parts are more strictly connected together, than those of any other philosophical hypothesis. Allow his principle, the universality of

gravity, and that it decreases as the squares of the distance increase, and all the appearances, which he joins together by it, necessarily follow...His system now prevails over all opposition...even I, while I have been endeavoring to represent all philosophical systems as mere inventions of the imagination...have insensibly been drawn in, to make use of language expressing the connecting principles of this one <u>as if they were the real chains</u> which nature makes use of to bind together her several operations....

Smith warned himself against misreading the invention of Newton's imagination as "the real chains" of nature. That warning has been amply justified by the radical transformations theoretical physics has undergone in our time. One of those radicals, Albert Einstein (1934) put it in these words: "To the discoverer...the constructions of his imagination appear so necessary and so natural that he is apt to treat them not as the creations of his own thought but as given realities."

This section on epistemology began with the sentence: "Science is a way of knowing, not a collection of facts." It ended with a warning against misreading "the inventions of ... imagination ... as if they were the real chains that nature makes use of to bind together her several operations...." Serious scientists, who think about epistemology, know those statements to be true; as a practical matter, they proceed from day to day as if theorems are real and as if today's "facts" are incontrovertible. The problem is magnified by the way science is taught to medical students. Lecturers focus on results rather than the history of the ideas and experiments that gave rise to the results on which practice is based. The psychological demands of clinical practice drive this process a step further. Distressed patients want to know "the diagnosis." Doctors find it uncomfortable to acknowledge when they do not know. Furthermore, there is an asymmetry to the blame attached to the failure to make a positive (i.e., "organic") diagnosis. An intern, who has "missed" a brain tumor or an infection, is much more heavily criticized than if he has overlooked the psychiatric diagnosis. As a result, doctors order repetitive, expensive, and sometimes hazardous tests in a vain effort to run down a "real" (that is, organic) condition, rather than accept a psychiatric explanation for the symptoms. Forty years ago, John Whitehorn (1961) proposed that the ability to deal with uncertainty should be central to medical education.

"The illusory expectation of certainty in knowledge, fostered by poor educational methods in science courses has inclined medical students and doctors to fight shy of the human aspects of medicine because, by such false criteria, it seems 'unscientific' – meaning unsatisfactorily deterministic and certain.... It is humanly difficult to weigh alternatives unless one can cultivate some tolerance of uncertainty.... A more reasonable awareness of uncertainty, a less dogmatic clinging to presumed certainties, a greater ability to face uncertainty with equanimity, a more generous and wiser sharing of leadership, ... might have done much to humanize medical leadership in the field of health care."
—Whitehorn 1961

Treating Disease and Treating Illness

We have measured 'quality of care' by determining whether the appropriate tests or treatments were ordered at the appropriate times, but these technologic appraisals do not reflect the quality of caring and things that are often most important to patients: communication, perception, reassurance, empathy, compassion (Alvan Feinstein).

That is why it is useful to distinguish between "disease" and "illness" (Eisenberg 1977). I reserve the term "disease" for the doctor's concept of sickness; and "illness" for the patient's experience of sickness. Physicians diagnose and treat diseases, which they conceive of as entities independent of subjectivity, rooted in abnormalities in bodily structure and function. By definition, a disease is the same wherever in the world it occurs, whatever beliefs may be held regarding its genesis or cure, and whomever it affects. The underlying pathology is verifiable by agreed upon "objective" methods.

Illness, in contrast to the biomedical definition of disease, is a social experience which occurs in the context of culture. When individuals experience discomfort or dysfunction, they are considered "ill" only when such manifestations are recognized as illnesses according to community standards. Of course, the impact of severe organ pathology on function or survival cannot be overruled by social consensus. But the victimized individual can lay claim to the prerogatives of patienthood and enter the pathways to cure only when the status of patienthood has been conferred by the community through its established mechanisms.

The biological events which underlie disease exist as phenomena in the world whether or not they are recognized. Their existence provides the occasion for their recognition. However, the identification of phenotypic variation as pathological is a social judgement. Consider the vicissitudes over time and space of a person suffering from pinta, known to western medicine as a disease caused by the spirochete *Treponema carateum*; it produces a variegated discoloration of the skin. Among North Amazonian Indians, the pigment disorder is so nearly universal that it is the unblemished, disease free individual who is labeled as deviant and excluded from marriage. Among the Aztec, those afflicted by pinta were selected by the Emperor Montezuma to bear his litter because their color complemented the display of his ornaments. In contemporary Mexico, "pintados" are shunned as disfigured (Ackerknecht 1946). Penicillin resolves pinta as a disease; changing community attitudes toward pintados is far more difficult a challenge to public health. CAM may comfort victims, but it is a poor third choice for the disease and illness of pinta.

Disease and illness do not run the same course; the extent of organ pathology does not correlate closely with patient distress; indeed, control of a disease may create the illness. Early in its course, hypertension is asymptomatic. Medication that succeeds in bringing the high blood pressure into the normal range sometimes produces stressing side effects. Some patients may give up on treatment altogether instead of returning to the physician for change in dose or in medication. Their "illness" (drug toxicity) remits, but their disease (hypertension) persists and carries with it the increased probability of a stroke. If a stroke does occur, the patient has both the disease and the illness, but available remedies can no longer fully restore health.

Conversely, ill patients seek help for epigastric pain. The physician will attribute the pain to ulcer disease if a crater can be visualized on endoscopy. The patient is placed on medication. If the crater heals over, the physician concludes that the patient is cured of the disease by definition. However, symptoms can persist when the ulcer disappears and may remit when the ulcer doesn't (Peterson et al. 1977). All too often, the physicians become dismissive of the complaints of the patients whose symptoms remain after "cure."

The goal of the healer should be to treat illness as well as disease.

For acute disease, cure of the disease cures the illness, surgery for appendicitis being a prototype. In chronic disease, cure may simply not be possible with a means currently at hand (arthritis, diabetes, metastatic cancer); illness management can, nonetheless, reduce distress and dysfunction. As suggested earlier, the very virtuosity of medical technology has caused physicians to narrow their interest to the diseased organ, cell, or molecule with a corresponding failure to appreciate the person in whom the pathological process occurs and to understand the family and community in which the patient lives. On the one side, this is driven by technology and on the other by economics. In a competitive medical marketplace, time becomes money, instead of being recognized as the essential ingredient of medical care. Demands to "process" patients more rapidly wreak havoc on the quality of care: time to listen, time to understand, time to educate, time to discuss the therapeutic options, and time for the patient to formulate his/her choice and to play an active role in treatment. To the degree that biomedicine fails to recognize and treat "illness," to that extent it increases the appeal of CAM.[v] As Alvan Feinstein (2000) has asked: "will the allopathic physicians continue to shun...unorthodox approaches, or will we recognize that they are often attractive because they offer patients the personal attention, concern and hope that they may not get from us?"

Randomized Controlled Trial as the Gold Standard

The scientific gold standard for clinical medical research is the double-blind, randomized, controlled trial (RCT). The purpose of "blinding" patients is to minimize the likelihood that the expectancy of good results aroused by the new therapy will produce symptomatic improvement in the absence of specific pharmacodynamic effects. The doctor is "blinded" because doctors undertake trials precisely because they expect the new treatment to be better. Expectation may lead the doctor to overread improvement in the experimentals and fail to see it in the controls, if he or she knows one from another. Treatment assignment can be subtly biased so that those with a better prognosis are preferentially assigned to the experimental group. It is not that experimenters are dishonest; it is precisely because they want to be honest that they turn themselves into neutral arbiters. Blinding can be difficult and it is sometimes impossible.

Random assignment begins only after patient eligibility for the trial has been determined. Does the patient meet diagnostic criteria for the disease? Is the patient willing and able to give informed consent? If there is reason to believe that gender, ethnicity, age, or other identified variables interact with either disease or treatment, patients may be stratified by these traits in order to ensure approximate balance before assignment is randomized. The purpose of randomization is not only to avoid bias, but to increase the probability that unknown variables will be distributed equally between the two groups by random assignment.

Bias arising from commercial interests is an increasing concern. Whereas ten years ago, 80 percent of drug trials were conducted by academic institutions, the not-for-profit share has dropped to 40 percent, and the majority of studies are conducted by for-profit research companies. In academia, trials may be carried out by investigators with stock in, or on a retainer from, pharmaceutical firms. What makes this worrying is that studies favoring their own drugs were reported 89 percent of the time in company-funded studies and only 61 percent among those funded form independent sources. Some firms deny researchers the right to publish unfavorable data. Data-analysis, and "ghost" or "guest" authors may be provided by the sponsor. The director-designate of the U.S. Office for Human Research Protection, Dr. Greg Koski, acknowledged "very real, very serious" problems in current research ethics, which constitute "a threat to our entire endeavor." It is his view (and mine!) that researchers should not conduct studies on products in which they own shares, a welcome public affirmation of an ethical position currently under great pressure.

What seems startling in retrospect is the recency of RCTs in medicine. Until the end of World War II, the justification for new treatments was provided by the opinions of senior clinicians who had tried the treatment on a series of patients and concluded that the outcome was better than that observed in the past. That approach worked well enough when the new treatment had dramatic effects, but it failed repeatedly when effects were small (or non-existent). It was gradually recognized that a system of concurrent controls was preferable and by the 1930s allocation of alternate patients to one or the other arm of the study was generally adopted. The system was flawed because physician judgment entered into patient allocation (Doll 1991). The first randomized control trial was the UK Medical Research Council (1948) trial of streptomycin for tuberculosis. Supplies of the drug were limited; it was known to be toxic. It was essential to establish effectiveness before release for wide-scale use. The investigators ruled out the use of placebo in the patients' interest; the controls would have had to receive intra-muscular injections four times a day for four months. Supplies did not permit the treatment of more than 50 patients, but the drug was so powerful that a highly significant reduction in mortality was evident after six months of observation.

The first RCT in pediatrics (Reese et al. 1952) was published four years later. It was a study of corticotropin treatment for retinopathy of prematurity (ROP). Newborns, screened for early signs of ROP, were put on corticotropin if signs were positive. The clinical investigators were under pressure to publish their promising early results, but worried about side effects and long-term hazards. They undertook a formal randomized trial; to their dismay, they found outcome better in the untreated controls because treated infants had more fatal infections. Thus, the first RCT in medicine demonstrated the effectiveness of a drug that proved to be instrumental in tuberculosis control; the first RCT in pediatrics stopped the diffusion into practice of a drug that would have had disastrous effects.

In some circumstances, only an RCT can detect the toxicity of a treatment with a logical rationale and visible effects. Dramatic events mislead clinicians. When ventricular arrhythmia reverts to normal rhythm during lidocaine administration, this registers on clinical consciousness as a treatment success; failure to respond is attributed to the underlying disease. Meta-analysis of RCTs conducted between 1970 and 1990 demonstrated that lidocaine was actually associated with a higher death rate (that is, it provoked as well as terminated arrhythmias) (Antman 1992).

Randomized trials sometimes seem to prove what doctors "knew" all along. But did they "know"? And "who" knew? Two RCTs of magnesium sulfate as a treatment for eclampsia (Eclampsia Trial Collaborative Group 1995) (Lucas et al 1995) in the UK and the US demonstrated the marked superiority of magnesium sulfate over diazepam and phenytoin in averting recurrent convulsions. Was this news? It wasn't "news" in the United States where magnesium sulfate had been the standard for 50 years; the findings flatly contradicted equally uniform but contrary practice in the UK where only 2 percent of obstetricians used it (Roberts 1995). In reality, neither group of doctors "knew;" both groups were guided by tradition.

Absent an RCT, the dispute was unresolvable.

In the half-century since their introduction, tens of thousands of RCTs have been carried out, more than two thousand of them trials on schizophrenia. Some were substantially flawed by one of more of the following: inadequate sample size, uncertain blinding, inconsistent methods of evaluation, too short a duration, or poor reporting (Thornley and Adams 1998). Nonetheless, in the aggregate they have improved the quality of patient care both by affirming the value of useful drugs and by halting the dissemination of toxic or ineffective ones.

The FDA requires proof of efficacy as well as safety before a new drug is allowed on the market. Unfortunately, RCTs are not required before technology is extended into new domains. A cogent argument for such a requirement is evident from a new medical market widely advertised on Internet and radio. Enterprising radiologists will provide on demand a computed tomography (CT) scan, magnetic resonance imaging (MRI) or a positron emission tomography (PET) scan for asymptomatic individuals worried that something somewhere may be wrong. CT scans, MRIs, and PETS are of unquestioned utility when deployed appropriately in medical diagnosis. But what is their predictive value when deployed on the general population? The predictive value of a positive finding depends not only on _sensitivity_, (i.e., the proportion of true cases who test positive) and its _specificity_ (the proportion of normal persons who test negative), but also on the _prevalence_ of the disease in the population being tested. Patients who consult the physicians are ordinarily referred for radiologic examination only if symptoms or physical findings suggest _a priori_ probability of disease. In a random population, prevalence of illness is far lower. Therefore, the ratio of false positives to true positives is necessarily much higher. At the least, the result will be increased anxiety until further examinations explain away the incorrect interpretation. But the workup itself may include invasive and risky tests, which may cause harm where no disease existed. Or the scan may indeed find an indolent tumor that might never have become symptomatic. Once found, it is treated at risk to the person who has become a patient (Eisenberg 1980).

One of the proponents of a "heart scan for calcium" in coronary arteries, Dr. Clouse of the Beth Israel Deaconess Medical Center, urges the procedure be done in all men over 40, even though there is no treatment for the condition. He argues that knowing that there are calcium deposits in coronary arteries will spur such individuals to make lifestyle changes. The fact that the American College of Cardiologists and the American Heart Association recommend against widespread screening has not altered his stance (Barnard 2000). What is needed is an RCT evaluating the impact of screening on health status; that is, does the benefit of detecting and removing asymptomatic lesions outweigh the negative health effects of false positives. Is profitability driving the market? The cost of a calcium scan is about 400 dollars and of a whole-body PET scan $3,500. Managed care, of course, won't pay on demand for scans; payment is out-of-pocket. There are no controls on the growth of this market except the extent to which consumers are educated by a cost/benefit analysis.

CAM and RCTs

How far can RCTs be employed to evaluate CAM? Herbal preparations can be tested against placebo in a classical RCT, but only if the active preparation can be standardized so that ingredients are the same from batch to batch. Acupuncture can be (and has been) tested by using pseudo needle points. "Magnet" therapy for back pain can be (and has been) tested by using metallic non-magnetized controls. However, difficulties in blinding and in random assignment limit the usefulness of RCTs for evaluating many CAM procedures. Random allocation to a "treatment" that a skeptical patient believes to be fraudulent or ineffective is obviously neither fair to the patient nor a fair test of such a therapy as faith healing. Even where blinding is not possible, comparative studies can be (and have been) undertaken to compare the treatment of chronic back pain by traction, bed rest, active exercise, chiropractic and other maneuvers (tincture of time seems to work about as well as any). The burden of proof should be on the "alternative" to prove itself when there are conventional treatments of established value. When there are not, all bets are off. When Samuel Hahnemann introduced homeopathy in the 19th century, part of the reason for its success must have been that the highly diluted "drugs" he recommended (some so highly diluted that not a molecule of the drug survived the serial dilutions!) had a big advantage over existing remedies (like purging and bleeding); they did no harm! They still do no harm; there is little evidence they do good; but taken in place of effective remedies, they put the patient at risk.

The Difference between Efficacy and Effectiveness

> We have determined the average efficacy of treatments from
> the results of randomized statistical trials, but the average
> results have not often been relevant to the clinical nuances
> of individual patients. We have agglomerated the results of
> multiple randomized trials into meta-analyses that are often
> called 'evidence-based medicine,' but what we need is a
> humanistic science containing medicine-based evidence.
> —Alvan Feinstein

The RCT remains an essential clinical research methodology. But it
is not the solution to all problems. The results of RCTs do not
always hold up in community practice. A case in point is the gap
between the percentage of depressed patients who improve on
drugs during RCTs in academic psychiatric settings and the often
mediocre results obtained in primary care practice (Eisenberg 1992).
What accounts for the slippage in translation from academia to daily
practice? That is, why is there a difference between "efficacy" and
"effectiveness"? Efficacy refers to a positive treatment result demonstrated in a rigorous RCT. Effectiveness refers to clinical outcomes
from the same treatment applied in the community under ordinary
conditions of practice. To what extent is the gap explained by differences between the research patient population and the practice
population? How far does the very fact of participating in a research
trial influence outcomes? To what extent is the difference due to a
lack of correspondence between the way treatment is provided in a
research clinic and in the practitioner's office?

Patient Samples

Patients who are included in a research trial must meet specified
diagnostic criteria. Those who do not meet threshold or have co-
morbidity are excluded. However, practitioners do not exclude
from care patients with sub-threshold diagnoses and co-morbidity.
Patients willing to be treated by a general practitioner may refuse
referral to a psychiatrist. Thus, the characteristics of the sample
reaching the psychiatric clinic are different from those treated in
general practice. Patients who do not acknowledge that they are
psychiatrically ill or who distrust "research" will not participate.

Participating in a new therapeutic enterprise may arouse expectations of benefit among participants. Although news stories regularly

portray subjects as "guinea pigs," the overall level of care provided in well designed clinical trials is, on average, better than that in random doctors' offices. Investigators study the patient in depth (in contrast to the pressure in a medical marketplace to get patients in and out); diagnosis is more precise; treatment is offered only to appropriate patients. Furthermore, clinical researchers have a heavy scientific investment in their patient subjects. Dropouts vitiate the validity of results. Therefore, investigators maximize convenient visit schedules, availability by telephone, and so convey interest to the patient. Just how powerful this can be is evident in the Diabetes Control and Complications Trial (1993). Despite a demanding treatment protocol and requirements for modifying lifestyle, 99 percent of the patients completed the 3-5 year trial, a tribute to the ability of the nurse-clinicians and dedicated investigators to build relations with patients.

Practitioner Skills

How much of the gap between efficacy and effectiveness is attributable to suboptimal practice? Implementation of protocol for the treatment of depression is often unsatisfactory; adherence is monitored poorly, if at all (Eisenberg 1992). Treatment compliance may differ markedly between the research sample and clinical practice. This goes a long way to account for poor results. Is the dose appropriate? Generalists often apply antidepressants in homeopathic doses. It is not enough to hand the prescription to the patient; the doctor must invest time and effort in explaining its utility, discussing its side effects, how long it will take before it works, and establishing with the patient criteria by which compliance will be measured. Compliance itself (whether to placebo or active drug) affects outcome and must be closely scrutinized (Coronary Project Group 1980).

Clinical trials of potent combination antiretroviral therapy have demonstrated rates of viral suppression below the limits of detection in as many as 95 percent of patients. Yet, rates reported from community settings are often well below the 50 percent range. The promise of treatment is not being achieved in many clinical settings. Medication adherence is the key variable. Adherence is affected by the program of clinical care, the characteristics of the professionals delivering that care, the treatment regimen, as well as by patient characteristics. "Blaming the patient" for failure of adherence is an unacceptable rationalization for inadequate care provision, at least until all measures to improve care have been tried and have failed (Reiter et al 2000).

Is there a "culture" of Western medicine?

> Human knowledge and human power meet in one; for
> where the cause is not known the effect can not be
> produced. Nature to be commanded must be obeyed,....
>   —Francis Bacon: *Novum Organum* (1620)

"Hard" scientists object to the formulation "culture of science." They
regard it as tantamount to equating their beliefs and practices with
those of a pre-scientific culture. But "culture" does not assume
homogeneity (i.e., all scientists do not share identical beliefs nor do
all Trobriand Islanders). Recognizing that biomedicine has a culture
of its own says nothing about the validity or invalidity of its beliefs.
A. L. Kroeber and Clyde Kluckhohn (1952) defined culture as

> patterns, explicit and implicit, of and for behavior acquired
> and transmitted by symbols, constituting the distinctive
> achievement of human groups, including their embodiments
> in artifact;... culture systems may, on the one hand, be con-
> sidered as products of action, on the other as conditioning
> elements of further action.

Science arises from the need of every community to know as much
as it can about the nature of the physical and biological world it
inhabits. Science is embedded in society; it is supported by it; science
changes society. Full-time practitioners of science did not emerge
until societies had resources sufficient to support differentiated
specialists. Scientific knowledge is power, even though scientists
may seek knowledge for its own sake. Curiosity is a wellspring of
scientific activity, but there are also rewards: prestige, income, and
job security. Originality in scientific discovery rewarded with prestige.
This makes priority a matter of pride, but it also leads to quarrels
over priority. Academic tenure has been the primary reward for
academic productivity since the early years of the last century. Pay,
on the other hand, was quite modest. Since World War II the dramatic
role of science in victory over fascism increased by an order of
magnitude academic salaries; in the past several decades, scientific
patents have made some scientists wealthy. The new economic
opportunities place the traditional values (openness and sharing
knowledge) under stress. Secrecy supersedes communication when
profitability takes center stage.

Is a Victory Possible for Either Side in the War?

It does not take a von Clausewitz to know that neither side in this war can conquer the other. The medical establishment mounts a therapeutic armamentarium of unparalleled effectiveness against life-threatening diseases. Complementary and alternative medicine relieve discomfort and suffering in chronic illnesses and somatization disorders. To the extent that physicians supplement their biomedical efficacy with sensitivity to, and skill in managing, psychosocial distress, patient satisfaction with medical care will improve and fewer patients will seek out alternatives.

However, the medical establishment will never succeed in eliminating CAM, despite the devout wishes of many of its adherents. Even if medical practice co-opts components of alternative medicine shown to be efficacious in clinical trials, many more herbs, procedures, and rituals than those which have been tested will continue in use. The elimination of all disease is an idle dream, no less absurd than the goal of curing all unhappiness. So long as there are sick patients who do not respond to medical care or are dissatisfied with their physicians or are unable to afford their fees, they will seek care from CAM practitioners. What is devoutly to be wished is that the quality of care delivered on both sides of this great divide will be improved by higher standards for licensure and close monitoring of the ethical behavior of all healers.

> As Feinstein (2000) puts it: The core principles [of medicine] are: (1) unswerving allegiance to always doing what's best for the patient; (2) continuing support for the basic biomedical research that produces new accomplishments; (3) vigorous development of the basic clinical-care research that produces a humanistic science for evaluating the accomplishments; and (4) restoration of the charitable caring that is called 'caritas'.

References

Abbott A. (2000) German fraud inquiry casts a wider net of suspicion. *Nature* 405:871-2.

Ackerknecht E.H. (1946) Natural diseases and rational treatment in primitive medicine. *Bulletin of the History of Medicine* 19:147-497.

Antman E. M., Lau J., Kupelnick B., Mosteller F., Chalmers T.C. (1992): A comparison of results of meta analyses of randomized control trials and recommendations of clinical experts: treatments for myocardial infarction. *JAMA* 268:240-8.

Balliett W. (2000) Review of Fraser C. God's Perfect Child: Living and Dying in the Christian Science Church. Metropolitan Books.

Barber B. (1968) The sociology of science. In Sills D. (Ed): International Encyclopedia of the Social Sciences. N. Y., MacMillan Co., vol.14:92-99.

Barnard A. (2000) Clinics market scans for the symptom free. *Boston Globe* August 26:A-1.

Beeson P.B. (1980) Changes in medical therapy during the past half-century. *Medicine* 59:79-99.

Bodenheimer T. (2000) Uneasy alliance: clinical investigators and the pharmaceutical industry. *NEJM* 243:1539-44.

Burton T.M. (1999) Surgery on the skull for chronic fatigue? Doctors are trying it. *Wall Street Journal.* November 11:A-1.

Buiatti E. et al. (1999) Results from a historical survey of the survival of cancer patients given DiBella multi-therapy. *Cancer* 86:2143-49.

Carstairs G.M., Kapur R.L. (1976) The Great Universe of Kota: Stress, Change and Mental Disorder in an Indian Village. Berkeley University of California Press.

Cohen M.L. (2000) Changing patterns of infectious disease. *Nature* 406:762-7.

Coronary Project Group (1980) Influence of adherence to treatment and response to cholesterol on mortality in the coronary drug project. *NEJM* 303:1038-41.

DCC Trial Research Group (1993) The effects of intensive treatment of diabetes on the development and progression of long-term complications in insulin-dependent diabetes mellitus. *NEJM* 329:977-86.

Dembner A. (2000) Internet hits pharmaceutical industry. *Boston Globe* Aug 16:A-5.

Dimsdale J. (1999) Wanted: hypothesis testing in alternative medicine. *Psychosomatic Medicine* 61:1-2.

Doll R. (1991) Development of controlled trials in preventive and therapeutic medicine. *Journal of Biosocial Science* 23:365-78.

Druss B.G., Rosenheck RA (1999) Association between the use of unconventional therapies and conventional medical services. *JAMA* 282:651-56.

Eclampsia Trial Collaborative Group (1995) Which anti-convulsive for women with eclampsia? Evidence from the Collaborative Eclampsia Trial. *Lancet* 355-63.

Eddleston M., Rajapakse S., Rajakanthan et al. (2000) Anti-digoxin FAB fragments in cardiotoxicity induced by ingestion of yellow oleander. *Lancet* 355:967-72.

Editorial (2000) When primum non nocere fails. *Lancet* 355:2007.

Einstein A. (1934). On the method of theoretical physics. *Philosophy of Science* 1:162.

Eisenberg D.M., Davis R.B., Ettner S.L. et al. (1998) Trends in alternative medicine use in the US, 1900-1997: Results of a follow-up national study. *JAMA* 280:1569-75.

Eisenberg L. (1977) Disease and Illness: Distinctions between professional and popular ideas of sickness. *Culture, Medicine, and Psychiatry* 1:9-23.

Eisenberg L. (1980) What makes persons "patients" and patients "well"? *American Journal of Medicine* 69:277-86.

Eisenberg L. (1981) The physician as interpreter: ascribing meaning to the illness experience. *Comprehensive Psychiatry* 22:239-48.

Eisenberg L. (1997) The social imperatives of medical research. *Science* 198: 1105-1110.

Eisenberg L. (1999) Whatever happened to the faculty on the way to the forum? *Annals of Internal Medicine* 159:2251-56.

Ernst E. (2000) Prevalence of use of complementary/alternative medicine: A systematic review. *Bulletin of the World Health Organization* 78:252-7.

Feinstein AR (2000) New worlds and old traditions. *The Pharos* Summer: 4-8.

Flexner A. (1910) Medical Education in the United States and Canada. Reprinted by Science and Health Publication, Washington, DC.

Fugh-Berman A. (2000) Herb-drug interaction. *Lancet* 355:134-38.

Glanz J. (2000) New tactic in physics: Hiding the answer. *New York Times*: Aug 13:D-1.

Hart J.T., Dieppe P (1996) Caring effects. *Lancet* 347:1606-08.

Henderson L.J. (1935) Pareto's General's Sociology: A Physician's Interpretation. Cambridge, Harvard University Press.

Henderson L.J. (1936) The practice of medicine as applied sociology. *Transactions of the Association of American Physicians* 51:8-22.

Hilts P.J. (2000) Medical research official cites ethics woes. *New York Times*, Aug 17:A-27.

Holton G. (1998) The Scientific Imagination. Cambridge, Harvard University Press.

Horton R. (1967) African traditional thought and western science. *Africa* 37:50-71,155-187.

Howell J.D. (1999) The paradox of osteopathy. *NEJM* 341:1465-8.

Kershaw S. (2000) City shuts illegal clinic that catered to Chinese. *New York Times*, Aug 17:A-27.

Kessler, D.A. (2000) Cancer and herbs. *NEJM* 342:1742-3.

Kroeber A., Cluckhohn C (1952, 1963) Culture: A Critical Review of Concepts and Definitions. New York, Vintage Paperbacks.

La Perla R. (2000) Hospitals discover their inner spa. *New York Times*. Aug 13:D-1

Lindenbaum, S. (1979) Kuru Sorcery: Disease and Danger in the New Guinea Highland. Palo Alto, Mayfield Publishing Company

Lucas M.J., Levine K.J., Cunningham F.G. (1995) The comparison of magnesium sulfate with phenytoin for the prevention of eclampsia. *NEJM* 333:201-5.

Medical Research Council (19848) Streptomycin treatment of pulmonary tuberculosis. *British Medical Journal* 2:769-82.

Middleton W.S. (1928) The Yellow Fever Epidemic of 1793 in Philadelphia. *Annals of Medical History* 10:434-450.

Mohr J.C. (2000) American medical malpractice litigation in historical perspective. *JAMA* 283: 1731-37.

Needham J. (1981) Science in Traditional China: A Comparative Perspective. Cambridge, Ma.: Harvard University Press.

Nortier, J.L., Muniz MC, Schmeiser HH, et al. (2000) Urothelial carcinoma associated with the use of the Chinese herb (Aristolochia fangchi). NEJM 342:1686-92.

Peabody F.W. (1930) Doctor and Patient. New York, MacMillan.

Peterson W.L., Sturdevant RAL, Frank HD et al. (1977) Healing of duodenal ulcer with an antacid regimen. NEJM 297:341-5.

Redfield R. (1941) The Folk Culture of Yucatan. Chicago, University of Chicago Press.

Reese A.R., Blodi FC, Locke JC, Silverman WA, Day RL (1952) Results of the use of ACTH in the treatment of retrolental fibroplasia. AMA Archives of Ophthalmology 47:551-5.

Reiter G.S., Stewart K.E., Wojtusik L.L. (2000) Elements of success in HIV clinical care: Multiple interventions that promote adherence. Topics in HIV Medicine 8:21-30.

Richmond J.B. (1969) Currents in American Medicine. Cambridge, Harvard University Press.

Ringel E.W. (1998): The morality of cosmetic surgery for aging. The Archives of Dermatology 134:427-31.

Roberts J.M. (1995) Magnesium sulfate for pre-eclampsia and eclampsia. NEJM 333:250-1.

Silverman W.A. (1980) Retrolental Fibroplasia: A Modern Parable. New York, Grune and Stratton.

Smith O.W. (1948) Diethylstilbestrol in the prevention and treatment of complications of pregnancy. American Journal of Obstetrics and Gynecology 56:821-34.

Steinhauer J. (2000) For some New York immigrants, a vast alternative health care system, underground. New York Times, August 20:A-24.

Stokstad E. (2000) Stephen Straus's impossible job. Science 288:1568-70.

Thornley B., Adams C. (1998) Content and quality of 2000 controlled trials in schizophrenia over 50 years. British Medical Journal 317:1181-4.

Turner, V. (1975) Revelation and Divination in Ndembu Ritual. Ithaca, Cornell University Press (pp 241-2).

Weiss R.B., Rifkin R.M., Stewart F.M. et al. (2000) High-dose chemotherapy for high-risk primary breast cancer: an on-site review of the Bezwoda study. Lancet 355:999-1003.

Wetzel M.S., Eisenberg D.M., Kaptchuk T.J. (1998) Courses involving complementary and alternative medicine at US medical schools. JAMA 280:784-87.

Whitehorn J.C. (1961) Education for uncertainty. NEJM 265:301-09.

Young, A. (1976) Some Implications of Medical Beliefs and Practices for Social Anthropology. American Anthropologist 78: 5-24.

Footnotes

I   Although alternative/complementary medicine is used at this conference as a single category to be contrasted with allopathic medicine or biomedicine or the "medical establishment", the terms "alternative" and "complementary" carry different implications. Complementary medicine is most appropriately used for health practices that supplement rather than replace Western medicine. Allopathic physicians may recommend or prescribe complementary treatments such as massage, acupuncture, special diets, exercise, etc. Alternative medicine should be limited to health practices employed in place of Western medicine (herbal remedies or macrobiotic diets instead of cancer chemotherapy). The distinction has much to do with the instructions given by individual healers as it does with the tenets of the healing system. In some surveys, as many as one in three adult Puerto Ricans consult spiritist mediums to diagnose and treat distress, particularly instances of psychological distress, interpersonal problems and chronic disease. Some spiritists refer their clients to physicians for additional consultation; they acknowledge that there are material, as well as spiritual, causes of illness and encourage their clients to cooperate with medical regimes. Others, however, interdict the use of Western medicines during spiritist treatment. Thus, spiritism may be "complementary" or "alternative" depending on how eclectic or how orthodox the practitioner is.

What is CAM today may be conventional tomorrow. When Andrew Taylor Still founded a school in 1892 to teach his system of osteopathy (manipulation of the spine to improve blood flow and allow the body "to heal itself,") it was in opposition to allopathic medicine which fought it all the way. But as osteopathic schools incorporated drugs and surgery and as medical associations became wary of court suits alleging restraint of trade, a move toward assimilation began in California in the 1960s. Eighty-six percent of the DOs in the state opted for an offer to trade in a DO for an MD degree. A majority of graduates of osteopathic schools choose allopathic residency training. The training of DOs resembles that of MDs more and more closely. Osteopathy, which began as "alternative," is no longer so. Chiropractic, founded at about the same time by Daniel David Palmer, is still CAM and mostly limited to spinal manipulation for chronic back pain. But its services are covered more and more often by third party payers.

II Complaints about practitioners being "too scientific" date from well before applied science had any appreciable impact on medical practice. Professor Francis W. Peabody wrote in 1923:

> The layman of the older generation... who feels that something has been lacking in the way of warmth, sympathy and understanding... is very apt to hark back to earlier days. 'What we need,' he says, 'is a general practitioner!

III Few, if any, of the participants in this meeting can claim to be unarmed, neutral civilians in the war between complementary/alternative medicine and the medical establishment. The best each of us can do is to acknowledge our sources of bias as honestly as we can. I have no stock in Harvard Medical School (no one does); as an emeritus professor, I do have a stake in its reputation (which reflects on me) and its endowment (on which my pension depends). However, since it would take a rather sizeable assault on reputation and endowment to reduce my modest pension, monetary considerations would hardly seem to matter. A more important source of bias is a fifty-year academic career. By definition, I am a member of the medical establishment (however uncomfortable I find it to acknowledge that fact). What matters still more are my intellectual convictions. Let me be up front about them. In my view, the best that the claims of CAM warrant is the Scot's verdict of "not proven." When put to the test with appropriate controls, most don't stand up. CAM theories, for the most part, defy what we know about the world (for example, claims for healing at a distance without attenuation). That, however, does not prove that CAM does not bring relief to some patients who seek it or that some healers do better than others. Those are empirical questions. Nor would I deny that some herbal remedies contain pharmacologically active drugs. Digitalis, quinine, ephedrine, and reserpine were all derived from folk remedies. Without doubt, other potent drugs remain to be identified. The yield, in my opinion, is likely to be low.

IV Most patients are pragmatists, willing to consult, either simultaneously or in succession, a series of healers with divergent methods. In an epidemiologic study of the village of Kota in India, Carstairs and Kapur (1976) identified 3 major types of healers in addition to Western trained physicians who served the population. The Vaids, practitioners of Ayurveda, ascribe illness to an imbalance between the natural elements, leading to an excess of heat, cold, bile, wind or fluid secretions which can be caused by such things as eating wrong food or uninhibited sexual indulgence; at the same time, disease can be caused by pisachis or evil spirits; treatment is by herbs, roots and pills. Mantarwadis are masters of the Zodiac and of potent secret verses termed mantras; cause is discovered through the Zodiac and cure is carried out through the mantra. The Patris act as mediums for a spirit or Bhuta which uses the healer's body and voice as a means of communicating to the patient the ways of exorcising evil. A survey of the population revealed that although Western practitioners were used as the sole source (40 percent) more often than indigenous healers (only 14 percent), the most common pattern of patient care was to employ both simultaneously (46 percent).

V As long ago as 1935, L. J. Henderson, professor of Biological Chemistry at Harvard Medical School [the Henderson of the Henderson-Hasselbach equation (a formula for the pH of a buffer solution: $pH = pk' + log(BA)/HA \times (HA))$], lamented the fact that the accomplishments of laboratory science had defeated the advocates of clinical instruction and resulted in a condition:

> in which the patient is... often a mere case, which (not who) passes through his doctor's office, his past, present, and future unknown, except with the meager abstractions of etiology, diagnosis and prognosis; and his personality and relations with other persons not even thought of.

Henderson enjoined physicians to remember that "a physician and a patient taken together make up a social system. In any social system, the interaction of the sentiments is likely to be at least as important as anything else." The physician-patient social system is almost a trivial one compared with the larger social system of which the patient is a permanent member and in which he lives. This system, indeed, makes up the greater part of the environment in which he feels that he lives. I suggest that it is impossible to understand any man as a person without knowledge of this environment and especially of what he thinks and feels it is; which may be a very different thing.

Henderson's pleas were entirely ineffectual. No remnant remains. But what he wrote is as true now as it was 70 years ago.

The Placebo Effect

Alvan R. Feinstein, M.D.
Yale University School of Medicine

Many people today have increasingly sought help, and believe they have received it, from unorthodox healing activities that may be called alternative, complementary, or fringe therapy. The orthodox medical reaction to these activities is sometimes to denounce them as "quackery", and more often to claim that the successes are merely a "placebo effect".

The denunciations and successes have brought new attention to the question, discussed [1-13] for more than half a century: "What is the placebo effect?" It is usually regarded as a single phenomenon produced by administration of an inert agent, but the effect actually arises from several factors that can alter a person's responses to treatment.

Contributions to Post-Theraputic Response

Beyond the specific action of the therapeutic agent itself, a person's post-therapeutic response can be affected by the phenomena of natural course, iatrotherapy, psychic state, and expectation.

1. Natural Course

Any ailment that occurs in the human body will have a natural biologic course of events, regardless of therapy. This course may or may not be favorable, according to the ailment and its host. The host's underlying condition may be such that an appropriate stimulus produces allergic or other adverse effects; but most often the body has its own beneficent biologic powers of healing. Many years ago, this power was given the Latin name, *vis medicatrix naturae*—the healing force of nature.

This natural capacity for healing is readily evident after acute ailments, such as a superficial cut or skin abrasion, a common cold, or recovery from a small stroke. The natural capacity can also alter the conditions of progression or alleviation for chronic illness, such as osteoarthritis or gallstones.

The role of nature (or of divinity) in healing was recognized many centuries ago by the French surgeon, Ambroise Paré, who said, "I dressed the wound. God healed it." The role of nature was generally ignored, however, when most orthodox physicians used post hoc reasoning to credit a specific treatment for the subsequent effects. Thus, until the early 19th Century, many acute ailments that today would probably be called the common cold, "flu," or upper respiratory infection, were regularly treated successfully with such therapies as blood-letting, blistering, purging, and puking. These treatments began to be discredited when doctors started using comparative groups, and recognized the existence of self-limited disease.

The role of natural healing still occurs today, of course. In the absence of controlled comparisons, however, it may be neglected; and post hoc reasoning may give credit for the improvement to whatever treatment — orthodox or unorthodox — was given to the patient. If the treatment happened to be an overt placebo, the response might be erroneously called "placebo effect."

2. Iatrotherapy

Beyond giving the actual therapeutic agent itself, the things that a therapist perceives, says, and does, with vocal or other communication, can have a powerful impact on good (or bad) results for the patient. The therapist's understanding, optimism, and reassurance are often dismissed as being merely "bedside manner." Nevertheless, this personal form of iatrotherapy can be a powerful and effective therapeutic agent. [14, 15]

Although iatrotherapy alone may make patients feel better, the favorable response may then be fallaciously deemed "placebo effect." The ability to produce this response, however, is a vital skill of good physicians. Blau [16] has suggested that "the doctor who fails to have a placebo effect on his patients should become a pathologist." I once made rounds with a famous surgeon who would pop his head in the patient's doorway for a moment, say a few pleasant words, and then depart. Many patients afterwards would state: "It makes me feel better just to see him."

For many physicians and other healers, the perception, attention, compassion, and other attributes of iatrotherapy are not easy to give — since they may require substantial personal effort— and they may be evoked only if the healer has faith in the effectiveness of the treatment. For example, a homeopathic physician I met several years ago had a magnificent personality that must have made her a splendid healer and a highly effective iatrotherapist. When I asked her, however, about the possible action of homeopathic solutions so dilute that they could not contain a single molecule of the original substance, she replied, "If I did not believe in the power of my medications, I could not give of myself."

3. Psychic State

Although purely biologic responses occur in the body, an ailment is also affected by the psychic state of the patient. According to that state, one person with a common cold will keep working; another will take to bed. One person with a sprained ankle will keep walking unaided; another will use crutches. Exactly the same pain stimulus may be accepted stoically as negligible or mild by one recipient, but regarded as severe or debilitating by another.

A person's psychic state, which includes cultural and religious background, can also profoundly affect individual beliefs about the cause and therapy of an ailment. These beliefs are apparent when people think either that their illness arises internally as punishment for a particular personal malefaction, or that the source is external, provoked by the curse or other evil intent of an enemy. Treatment may then succeed or fail according to how well it corresponds to the patient's underlying belief about pathogenesis. A more modern form of psychic pathogenesis and therapy may occur in the post-auto-accident whiplash syndrome, which can defy diverse therapeutic efforts for many months until the symptoms subside as soon as the lawsuit is settled.

4. Expectation

Beyond the direct effects and reactions of the psyche, people can have a sense of relief or satisfaction merely because they have made the decision to seek and receive help. Sometimes they feel better because of favorable expectations produced by the reputation of a particular therapist or therapy. The therapist's expectation that a particular treatment will be effective may also evoke the iatrotherapy discussed previously.

Suggestibility, conditioning, and expectations can also affect the way that both doctors and patients respond to individual stimuli.[10] The expectation that produces "placebo-reactor" effects in physicians can alter not only their positive or negative approaches to therapy, but even their diagnostic interpretations. Radiologists have been found to change their opinions about the interpretation of images when given a deliberately false history that suggested findings contrary to what was in the film.[17] In patients, the previously demonstrated efficacy of a drug declined when they were told of the possiblity that it might be placebo.[18] Changes in size or color of the capsule may evoke different effects with the same oral medication. Nausea and vomiting can develop more often if recipients of the same medication are warned to expect those side effects than when given no anticipatory information.

To deal with the negative effects of expectation, the name nocebo [19] has been proposed for something that is like a placebo in being essentially inert or harmless, but that is perceived as harmful, and followed by an adverse impact. Nocebo events can occur as individual phenomena, but can also affect groups, with results that produce epidemics of hysteria.[20] Such epidemics have occurred, for example, when school children or other groups were exposed to odors that were believed noxious, but that actually were not.

Expectation can also be applied improperly by house staff and nurses. They may give placebos, instead of active medication, to patients who are disliked [21] when suspected of malingering, exaggerating their pain, or otherwise being "undeserving". A favorable response to the placebo, which might very well occur as a true "placebo effect," is then regarded as confirmation of the patient's unworthiness. Practicing physicians seldom use overt placebos, but often prescribe agents that might possibly be effective — such as Vitamin B-12 for fatigue or antibiotics for viral ailments — as a way of satisfying a patient's expectation or psychic need for therapy, and also perhaps to shorten the office visit.

Many years ago, working as an obesitologist, I spent about an hour, with someone who wanted to reduce her substantial overweight, explaining various facts of nutrition and calories, and prescribing an appropriate dietary regimen. After I finished the instructions, she expressed surprise that I was not giving her an injection; and she vehemently asked for one, saying, "I never lose weight without injections." I repeated the discussion, assured her that she did not need an injection, and would lose weight simply by maintaining the proposed regimen. She kept insisting she needed the injection, and I kept insisting she did not. Finally, to end the argument, I said, "Very well. I will give you an injection, but it will be salt water."

She happily accepted it, and returned two weeks later, having followed the diet and lost five pounds. "I told you," she said triumphantly, "that I need injections to lose weight."

In an era of high technology, the benefits of expectation can sometimes be evoked by diagnostic rather than therapeutic procedures. For example, an occasional patient with the irritable colon (or functional bowel distress) syndrome, not fully understanding the sequential medical events in care, may report major improvement after the barium enema or colonoscopy that was part of the diagnostic "workup". Other impressive technical procedures that are done not for therapy but for diagnosis, such as a computerized tomographic (CT) scan or magnetic resonance imaging (MRI), may also be followed by reports of substantial improvement in whatever ailment was being investigated.

5. Specific Action

Since natural healing, iatrotherapy, psychic effects, and expectation can all occur regardless of the type of preceding therapy, the specific action of a therapeutic agent is usually regarded as the treatment. The agent may lower blood pressure, blood sugar, or blood lipids; it may lyse thrombi, prevent clotting, kill bacteria, destroy cancer cells, alter mood, or affect the levels of various hormones.

The scientific basis of orthodox medical practice today consists of documentary evidence for these specific actions. One type of evidence comes from of laboratory (and sometimes clinical) experiments, that produce pharmacologic or pathophysiologic data to explain the agents' mechanisms of action. A second type of evidence, derived from randomized trials or other pertinent post-therapeutic observational studies, demonstrates the agent's clinical superiority when compared against other agents, no treatment, or a presumably inert substance, called placebo.

All types of healers, using orthodox or unorthodox types of treatment, will offer explanations for what a treatment does and why it works. For example, for many centuries orthodox physicians believed in the humoral theory of illness, which attributed ailments to imbalances in the four humors of blood, phlegm, yellow bile, and black bile. The treatments with various forms of blood letting, blistering, purging, and puking were intended to rectify the humoral imbalances. In orthodox medicine, the humoral theory began to go out of fashion about two centuries ago with the advent of autopsies and laboratory research. Humoral theories still persist, however, in certain forms of traditional medicine in Asia; and many analogous theories — based on substances, channels, and other pathways that have never been actually isolated or demonstrated — still exist in unorthodox forms of medicine.

Probably the main feature that distinguishes orthodox and unorthodox medical practice today is documentary evidence for the mechanisms of specific action and the efficacy of therapy. The results and ideas may sometimes turn out to be wrong; and the old concepts become replaced with new ones, such as the recent etiologic evidence that has led antibiotics to replace anti-acid treatment for peptic ulcer. Research efforts have even been made to demonstrate a mechanism of action for the "placebo effect" in analgesia. The claim that placebos lead to release of endorphins, however, has been contradicted, [22-25] and is currently still controversial. The persons who practice or do research in orthodox medicine usually realize that they may not always be right, but they now have a well-established tradition of checking to find and correct errors. This tradition has not yet become established in unorthodox forms of healing.

Types of Comparison

As a major accomplishment of modern orthodox medical science, randomized clinical trials are often intended to distinguish the effects of the fifth component of healing (specific action) from the first four contributions (nature, iatrotherapy, psyche, and expectation), which can be subsumed in the single phrase, "placebo effect." The choice and method of administration of the comparative agent in clinical trials depend on the contributions to be distinguished.

Methods of comparison

If an effective active agent has already been documented, it usually becomes used as the comparison or "control". For example, the merits of a surgical bypass operation for coronary disease may be compared against known effective agents, such as various forms of medical therapy or angioplasty. On the other hand, in trials of screening for breast cancer or colon cancer, where no other "effective" agent has been demonstrated, the comparison is against no screening.

For new pharmaceutical agents, a "no-treatment" comparison is seldom desirable, because the treated group will be affected by both the expectation and iatrotherapy that are lacking in the untreated patients. Consequently, the comparative agent for pharmaceutical trials is either some other active agent or a placebo.

The compared pharmaceutical agents are usually prepared to look and seem the same. This similarity produces the "double blinding" that is believed to keep both the therapist and the patient unaware of the treatment being given. This type of blinding is particularly important for comparisons against placebo, where knowledge that a treatment is placebo may lead to unfavorable expectations by the patient and failure by the clinician to offer enthusiastic iatrotherapy. This enthusiasm, of course, may be less in a placebo-controlled trial than in regular practice, because the clinician knows that the patient in the trial may have only a 50:50 chance of getting the "active" agent.

A tricky problem in choosing a comparative treatment arises when a new pharmaceutical agent is tested in circumstances where many alternative active agents are available. Rather than choosing one of those active agents (and then risking complaints that the most appropriate one was not chosen), the investigator and the FDA may prefer a "standardized" test of efficacy, for which the comparative agent is placebo.

For example, suppose I have developed a new drug, Excellitol, for treatment of hypertension. The drug seems to be wonderful: it lowers blood pressure gently but firmly; it has no substantial effects on potassium or other metabolites; and it does magnificent things for libido — raising libido if it needs raising and lowering it if it is too high. I now want to show the efficacy of Excellitol in randomized trials. Of the many single agents and combinations of agents that are available for treating hypertension, which one do I chose for comparison? If I choose A, someone will complain that I should have chosen B or C. If I choose B or C, someone else will argue that I should have chosen D or E. No matter what I choose, complaints will come that I did the wrong comparison.

With this dilemma, I realize that I have another prime goal: to get Excellitol approved by the FDA. When I check with the FDA, however, they tell me to use placebo.[26] It is a "standardized" agent; it avoids the problem of which other active agent to choose; and the results found with the placebo comparison can readily be contrasted and evaluated against the results of other agents that were also compared against placebo.

Ethical Problems

This approach will solve my challenge in finding a comparison, and the FDA will have done its duty as a regulatory agency, but they and I may then be accused of being unethical, because the persons receiving placebo were denied an effective treatment.[25] As an extreme example of this problem, in one long-term trial in Germany, the mortality rate was found to be higher with placebo than with the active drug. The investigators who gave the placebo regimen were then denounced, by a professor of law, as being "guilty of manslaughter".[28]

Whether we compare two active treatments, or an active treatment vs. placebo, the double-blinding is needed to avoid the problems of "placebo effect", creating unequal expectations and iatrotherapy in the compared groups. Double-blinding (which ophthalmologists and other investigators prefer to call "double-masking") also has major clinical and scientific advantages, however, beyond a mere avoidance of the "placebo effect."

For example, when the first large-scale trial was being done to test a vaccine against poliomyelitis, physicians might have felt unethical about letting their patients receive an overt placebo, particularly if the vaccine was later found to be effective. Double-blinding helped remove this possible guilt and reluctance to participate. The double-blinding also has an advantage in recruiting patients for a trial. After admission to an "unblinded" study, patients may be unwilling to continue if they discover that they have been assigned to placebo. During the course of the trial itself, a knowledge of the main treatment can bias the way the physician evaluates various manifestations and orders additional tests or therapy. Finally, at the outcome end of the trial, the appraisal of subjective phenomena, such as relief of symptoms or performance of various daily functions, can also be substantially biased by a knowledge of the prior treatment.

For all these reasons, double-blinding of the compared treatments is regarded as a highly desirable or essential procedure in evaluating therapy. The double-blinding process is relatively easy for oral pharmaceutical agents, since we can readily make one capsule or tablet look like another. The double-blinding may not always be effective, however. Certain active agents may be distinguished from placebo because of a concomitant physiologic effect, such as bradycardia, that can occur with beta blockers. Sometimes the recipients may bite into the capsule and taste the agent — an event that happened when staff working at the NIH were the subjects of a trial comparing Vitamin C with placebo in preventing colds. Patients can also use unorthodox methods of detection. In one apocryphal story, a patient in a cross-over trial is said to have asked the doctor, "Did you change my medication two weeks ago?" "Why do you ask?" replied the surprised doctor. "Well," was the response, "when I threw the previous pills into the toilet, they promptly sank. The new pills float."

A tricky problem in getting suitable double-blind comparisons occurs when the active treatment is inserted subcutaneously, as with acupuncture. The "placebo" control may consist of inserting acupuncture needles either to the wrong "depth" or in places different from the correct theoretical locations.

If an active oral agent is compared with an active injected substance, the activities needed to achieve double-blinding can lead to separate problems in ethics. The double-blinding would require that the persons getting the active injection also be given an oral placebo and that those receiving the active oral agent also get an injected placebo. Aside from the difficulty of maintaining a truly double-blind arrangement for the combined injection-oral program, one of the potential ethical problems is that half of the patients will have received unnecessary injections. Another problem, which is perhaps more clinico-scientific than ethical, is that the trial will not correspond to reality in clinical practice. Whatever regimen is superior in the trial will not be used that way by practitioners, who may give future patients either the better oral agent or the injection, but not a combination of active and placebo agents.

Sham Therapy

A particularly difficult ethical problem is to get a suitably "blind" comparison when the active treatment is a surgical procedure. The only thing that can be suitably "blinded" for comparison is another surgical procedure — done in the same way, but as a "sham." This tactic was used in two small randomized trials about 40 years ago [29,30] when ligation of the internal mammary artery, by presumably increasing coronary blood supply, had become a popular treatment for relieving angina pectoris. In the clinical trial, after the patients were suitably prepared and anesthetized in the operating room, a ligature was passed around the internal mammary artery. The surgeon then opened a sealed, sterilized opaque envelope containing the randomized instruction: TIE IT or DON'T TIE IT. Subsequent examiners and the patient were kept unaware of what had been done. When the doubly blinded outcome results showed that about 70 percent of the patients had improved in each of the ligated and sham groups, the operation was soon abandoned.

These trials today would be deemed unethical because the patients had not given a completely informed consent. Even with that consent, however, the trial might still be ethically condemned because the sham patients would be exposed to all of the hazards of a surgical procedure that presumably could not help them. Nevertheless, society was presumably benefited by the elimination of an operation that was no better than a sham. In addition, an extra benefit, which might not have happened without the real or sham surgery, occurred in the 70 percent of patients who improved.

This problem has reappeared today in the treatment of severe Parkinsonism, when stem cells are surgically implanted into the brain, with a sham procedure being used in the control group. Despite the ethical conflicts, the sham surgery seems to be the only way for patients, doctors, and society to determine whether the operation's benefits are worth its substantial risks and costs.

Improvements from Clinimetrics

The frequency of these problems could be substantially reduced with better observational studies of the events that occur under customary clinical conditions and in the initial introduction of new therapy. My colleagues and I have been advocating an improved observational approach for more than a decade,[31,32] but we have had only minimal success in getting acceptance from the "establishment." Nevertheless, with suitable criteria for selecting appropriate comparison groups (sometimes called "refined cohorts"), the results of several pertinent observational studies were found to be similar to those of the corresponding randomized trials.

With better clinimetric measures[33] to identify often neglected details of baseline conditions, such as clinical severity, the comparative groups could be made more similar for evaluating treatments. If outcome events also had better clinimetric identification — such as asking patients whether they are better and the reasons why they feel better (or worse) — double-blinding might not be needed as frequently as it is used today. Instead of talking carefully to patients, however, clinicians and investigators may apply multi-item psychometric measurements, which are deemed "reliable' and "valid", but which often fail to detect some of the most important subjective distinctions. [34]

Unfortunately, the proposed improvements in clinical observation are not likely to occur soon. They may begin to happen in the future, however, when defects in the current paradigms about randomization, double-blinding, psychometric instruments, and placebo controls have become more prominent and more susceptible to desirable changes.

Effects of Compliance

An activity that is sometimes erroneously confused with "placebo effect" is compliance — the patient's fidelity in taking (or "adhering to") an assigned therapeutic regimen. Perceptive clinicians have always known that patients may not take their medications faithfully, but the concept of "compliance" did not become formally recognized and labelled until the advent of campaigns against hypertension. When blood pressure did not adequately respond to treatment, many doctors ruefully discovered that the therapeutic agent had failed to work not because it was ineffective, but because it had not been taken. After the enlightenment of a discovery that should have been relatively obvious, compliance became another entity to be measured in clinical trials.

In one famous trial — the Coronary Drug Project (CDP) [35] — the investigators were surprised to find that a presumably active lipid-lowering agent had results no better than placebo in treating patients with coronary disease. The results in the group receiving the active agent were therefore partitioned and found to be much better in patients who had complied well than in those who complied poorly. The apparent superiority seemed to confirm that the active agent was indeed effective, until similarly superior results were noted in the placebo patients who had complied well rather than poorly.

The one entity that seemed to be unequivocally effective in the CDP trial was compliance. Instead of trying to determine the constituent elements of compliance and why it was effective, however, the clinical investigators and their statistical consultants interpreted the data to reach a different conclusion. They decided that, in the future, all clinical trials should be analyzed according to the regimens to which patients had been randomly assigned, not according to what the patients actually did afterward. This strategy, called the intention-to-treat policy, has now become another entrenched doctrine in the analysis of clinical trials. The strategy allegedly eliminates the bias that can be produced by differences in compliance (or by other events that occur after randomization), but it also eliminates many elements of clinical common sense. Someone randomly assigned to surgery and who then refuses it by taking only medical therapy is still counted as having had the surgery. Someone randomized to medical therapy but who decides to have surgery is counted as though he hadn't received it. What is most important to patients and doctors, of course, is not the statistical accolade of a randomized assignment, but what happens afterward. In the current statistical doctrines, however, the only thing to be considered is the randomized intention to give a treatment, not the treatment that was actually received.

Furthermore, if compliance is an important determinant of therapeutic outcome, we need to find out what determines the effect of compliance. Does the patient's psychic state predispose to both good compliance and a good outcome? Or is the good effect actually due to the ancillary (rather than the main) treatment taken by those who comply? With the prevailing statistical doctrine, however, we shall never find out. The sanctity of statistical randomization is regarded as more important than the sanity of clinical science.

Orthodox and Unorthodox Approaches

Both the orthodox and unorthodox branches of the healing arts can tell mutually antagonistic stories about their own successes after the other group's failures. The orthodox groups can regularly point to patients who died because of meningitis, hypoadrenalism, bleeding ulcer, or other major curable organic disease that had been unrecognized during ongoing treatment by unorthodox methods. The unorthodox groups can point to deaths from anaphylactic reactions or post-operative emboli in orthodox therapy, and to successful responses in patients with functional somatic syndromes[36] that had not responded to orthodox treatments. Instead of mutual hostility, however, the two groups might consider the possibility of mutual enlightenment or even collaboration. Both the orthodox and the unorthodox practitioners have much to learn from one another.

Opportunities for Orthodox Enlightenment

Instead of disdaining the "placebo effect," orthodox practitioners can become better doctors by making use of its components and contributions. More applications of iatrotherapy, and recognition of the roles of psyche and expectation, can help orthodox practitioners improve their work as healers in caring for patients. A major obstacle to this improvement today, however, is that "quality of care" is conceived and measured exclusively according to the use of authorized, approved technical procedures.[37] Such elements of care as comforting distress, providing reassurance, and alleviating anxiety are all components of good iatrotherapy — but they may not be taught well to medical students, exemplified to house staff, used by practitioners, or rewarded when audits of "quality of care" are confined solely to whatever specific procedures and medications were offered. With "quality of care" equated to the use of appropriate technology, and with the quality of "caring" ignored in orthodox medicine, patients may then be distressed by the absence of the humane iatrotherapy that comes from attention, empathy, and compassion. These attributes are often used, however, when treatment is given by unorthodox practitioners.

Furthermore, the customary forms of orthodox "allopathic" therapy regularly fail in two types of clinical situations. One of them is in patients with functional somatic syndromes[36] such as bowel distress, tension headaches, hyperventilation, fibromyalgia, and chronic fatigue syndrome. These ailments do not have the abnormalities of an "organic disease" and may respond poorly to diverse pharmaceutical agents. The other situation occurs with the incurable chronic ailments (metastatic cancer, neurologic disability) that are also not always helped by the available orthodox treatments. In all these circumstances, patients who feel they have received neither worthwhile help nor adequate hope may look elsewhere for aid from unorthodox sources.

Finally, a few of the unorthodox procedures may actually be effective and might be useful if learned by orthodox physicians. For example, chiropractic treatment has regularly produced relief for certain forms of low back pain. (My father used to tell me, "I go to your internist, and he gives me pills. Then I go to my chiropractor and he makes my back feel better"). Also, since orthodox medicine relied on botanical preparations for many centuries, we should not be surprised when efficacy is found today for certain herbal preparations, such as willow bark extract.[38]

On the other hand, orthodox therapists should be given credit for sometimes being remarkably flexible in meeting the psychic needs of patients from different cultures. I was present at an incident in Australia, about a decade ago, when an East Asian woman, although apparently cured by surgery, was highly distressed for a long time afterward because she believed her "soul spirit" had left her body during the operation. After various types of reassurance had failed, the surgeons returned the woman to the same operating room as before, gave her anesthesia, and then "found" and "returned" the missing entity. Afterward, the woman was delighted and achieved full recovery.

Opportunities for Unorthodox Enlightenment

For unorthodox forms of therapy, a major attraction is that the practitioners often take time to listen carefully to patients, and can thus be highly effective in using the roles of expectation, psyche, and iatrotherapy. In addition, when an ailment such as hysterical paralysis involves highly complex cultural or psychodynamic sources, the orthodox approaches of authoritative professors of neurology, neurosurgery, or even psychiatry may all be ineffectual. A surprising, dramatic unorthodox cure may then be achieved by a charismatic faith healer or a visit to the Shrine of Lourdes.

The major hazards of unorthodox therapy are the often unrecognized adverse effects of certain treatments (e.g., herbal agents, unsanitary acupuncture) and, most importantly, the failure to seek effective orthodox therapy in situations where it can be curative or life-saving. The practitioners of unorthodox therapy can avoid a great deal of criticism and recrimination if they would develop, teach, and use methods to recognize and refer such situations before major harm occurs.

Finally, unorthodox practitioners are also subject to the post hoc self delusion that attributes post-therapeutic success to the therapeutic agent. This delusion would not be a problem if the unorthodox treatments were always successful; but since they are not, the practitioners are challenged to determine which types of patients are particularly likely to be helped or not helped. This goal is difficult to attain in the absence of a distinctive nosologic or other form of diagnostic classification for the unorthodox concepts of ailments, and in the absence of enumerated results.

Several years ago, I asked a specialist in Chinese herbal therapy how she decided that a patient had an excess or deficit of liver xi, which is a fundamental principle in that form of treatment. I also wanted to know roughly how many patients she had treated with each form of her therapy, and how many of the courses of treatment had been successful. Her response was to explain the basic theory of action for liver xi, to urge me to spend a year with her to learn how to employ the therapy, and to state, somewhat scornfully, that she and her colleagues did not use western medical science. I replied that I was not requesting randomized trials or any elements of western medical science; I was just asking for some simple book-keeping. She then terminated the conversation, stating that I was too hopelessly biased for any further discussion.

The practitioners of unorthodox medicine probably have many good reasons for being paranoid about orthodox medicine. They can greatly help their own cause and that of their patients, however, by developing some simple systems of classification and tabulation. The unorthodox practitioners need not immediately proceed to ran-domized double-blind trials to demonstrate efficacy, and they need not institute laboratory studies of pathogenesis and therapeutic mechanisms, but they can certainly be expected and requested to provide some simple accounts of what kind of ailments are helped, what kind are not, and what is meant by "helped".

Conclusions

Both the orthodox and unorthodox practitioners have had many successes to make them proud, and many failures to keep them humble. They also have much to learn from one another. Orthodox medicine can benefit by making greater use of the iatrotherapy, expectation, and psychic reactions that are often dismissed as "placebo effect". Unorthodox medicine can benefit by recognizing the circumstances in which orthodox treatment is uniquely effica-cious or life-saving, and by getting better information about the particular circumstances in which unorthodox treatment can be uniquely helpful. Both groups want to be healers for their patients. A useful step toward that goal is to heal the current schism that keeps the two groups from being cooperative rather than antagonistic, and from making better use of each other's most effective approaches.

This conference contains some sessions on the value of teaching unorthodox methods to students in orthodox medicine. My own belief is that the instruction would be most valuable if it focused on the components of the "placebo effect" that accompanies unorthodox treatment, rather than on the explanatory theories and techniques of the unorthodox treatments themselves. Before the days of modern technologic advances, medical students learned about iatrotherapy, expectation, and psychic state during apprenticeships to physicians whose specific therapeutic agents would today be regarded mostly as ineffectual "placebos." Those older physicians, as exemplified in the famous painting by Luke Fildes, gave of themselves because they seldom had more to rely on. Today, however, with so much technologic splendor available, orthodox physicians may no longer appreciate or be taught the need to give of themselves. Unorthodox medicine can therefore be particularly helpful if it reminds or helps teach technocratic clinical scientists how to listen to patients and become better doctors and healers.

Postscript

Just as this manuscript was being sent to the printer, Drs. A. Hröbjartsson and P.C. Gøtzsche published a meta-analysis (NEJM; 344:1594-1602,2001) showing "little evidence in general that placebos had powerful clinical effects." This result is exactly what would be anticipated, because the "placebo effect,' as discussed in my comments, is not really an action attributable to the placebo itself. The "effect" is a post-therapeutic response arising from such therapeutic accompaniments as natural course, iatrotherapy, psychic state and expectation. These accompaniments can often lead to positive responses regardless of the particular agent, including placebo, that is used as the main therapy.
— A.R.F.

REFERENCES

1. Pepper, O.H.P. A note on the placebo. Tr. & Stud., Coll. Physicians, Philadelphia, 1945;13:81.
2. Findley, T. The placebo and the physician. M. Clin. North America 1953;37:1821.
3. Lasagna, L., Mosteller, F., von Felinger, J.M., Beecher, H.K. A study of the placebo response. Am. J. Med. 1954;16:770-779.
4. Leslie, A. Ethics and practice of placebo therapy. Am. J. Med 1954;16:854-862.
5. Beecher, H.K. The powerful placebo. JAMA 1955;159:1602-1606.

6. Joyce, C.R.B. Consistent differences in individual reactions to drugs and dummies. *Br. J. Pharmac.* 1959;14:512-521.

7. Wolf, S. The pharmacology of placebos. *Pharmacol. Rev.* 1959;11:689-704.

8. Shapiro, A.K. A contribution to a history of the placebo effect. *Behav. Sci.* 1960;5:109-135.

9. Benson, H., Epstein, M.D. The placebo effect: a neglected asset in the care of patients. *JAMA* 1975;232:1225-1227.

10. Byerly, H. Explaining and exploiting placebo effects. *Perspect. Biol. Med.* 1976; Spring: 423-436.

11. Brody, H. The lie that heals: the ethics of giving placebo. *Ann. Intern. Med.* 1982;97:112-118.

12. Gowdey, C.W. A guide to the pharmacology of placebos. *Can Med. Assoc.* J. 1983;128:921-925.

13. Spiro, H.M. Doctors, Patients, and Placebos. 1986. New Haven, Ct. Yale University Press.

14. Houston, W.R. The doctor himself as a therapeutic agent. *Ann. Int. Med.* 1938;11:1416.

15. Feinstein, A.R. Clinical Judgment. Baltimore. Williams & Wilkins Co. 1967.

16. Blau, J.N. Clinician and placebo. (Letter to Editor) *Lancet.* 1985;1:344.

17. Elmore, J.G., Wells, C.K., Howard, D.H., and Feinstein, A.R. The impact of clinical history on mammographic interpretations. *JAMA.* 1997;277: 49-52.

18. Skovlund, E. Should we tell trial patients that they might receive placebo? (Letter to Editor) *Lancet.* 1991;337:1041.

19. Schweiger, A., Parducci, A. Nocebo: the psychologic induction of pain. *Pavlov J. Biol. Sci.* 1981;16:140-143.

20. Boss, L.P. Epidemic hysteria: A review of the published literature. *Epidemiol. Rev.* 1997;19:223-243.

21. Goodwin, J.S., Goodwin, J.M., Vogel, A.V. Knowledge and use of placebos by house officers and nurses. *Ann. Int. Med.* 1979;91:106-110.

22. Levine, J.D., Gordon, N.C., Fields, H.L. The mechanism of placebo analgesia. *Lancet.* 1978;2:654-657.

23. Goldstein, A., Grevert, P. Placebo analgesia, endorphins, and naloxone. *Lancet.* 1978;ii:1385.

24. Gracely, R.H. Dugner, R., Wolskee, P.J., Deeter, W.R. Placebo and naloxone can alter postsurgical pain by separate mechanisms. *Nature.* 1983;306:264-265.

25. Grevert, P., Albert, L.H., Goldstein, A. Partial antagonism of placebo analgesia by naloxone. *Pain.* 1983;16:129-143.

26. Temple, R. Government viewpoint of clinical trials. *Drug Inform. J.* 1982;16:10-17.

27. Wilhelmson, L. Ethics of clinical trials — The use of placebo. *Eur. J. Clin. Pharmacol.* 1979;16:295-297.

28. Burkhardt, R., Kienle, G. Controlled clinical trials and medical ethics. *Lancet.* 1978;1356-1359.

29. Cobb, L.A., Thomas, G.I., Dillard, D.H., et al. An evaluation of internal-mammary-artery ligation by a double-blind technic. *N. Engl. J. Med.* 1959;160:1115-1118.

30. Dimond, E.G., Kittle, C.F., Crocket, J.E. Comparison of internal mammary artery ligation and sham operation for angina pectoris. *Am. J. Cardiol.* 1960;5:483-486.

31. Feinstein, A.R. Epidemiologic analyses of causation: the unlearned lessons of randomized trials. *J. Clin. Epidemiol.* 1989;42:481-489.

32. Concato J., Shah N., Horwitz R.I. Randomized controlled trials, observational studies, and the hierarchy of research designs. *New Eng. J. Med.* 2000;342:1887-1892.

33. Feinstein, A.R. Clinimetrics. 1987. New Haven. Yale University Press.

34. Feinstein, A.R. Multi-item "instruments" vs. Virginia Apgar's principles of clinimetrics. *Arch. Int. Med.* 1999;159:125-128.

35. Coronary Drug Project Research Group. Influence of adherence to treatment and response of cholesterol on mortality in the Coronary Drug Project. *N. Engl. J. Med.* 1980;303:1038.

36. Barsky, A.J. and Borus, J.F. Functional somatic syndromes. *Ann. Intern. Med.* 1999;130:910-921.

37. Feinstein, A.R. (Abstract) The mismeasurement of "quality of care". *J. Clin. Epidemiol.* 2000;53:438.

38. Chrubasik, S. Eisenberg, E., Balan, E., Weinberger, T., Luzzati, R. Conradt, C. Treatment of low back pain exacerbations with willow bark extract: A randomized double-blind study. *Am. J. Med.* 2000;109:9-14.

Survey of Complementary and Alternative Medicine Education

Miriam S. Wetzel, Ph.D.
Harvard Medical School

Now that the use of so-called Complementary and Alternative Medicine (CAM)* has become firmly established and clearly documented as a feature of the US health care scene,[1,2] the public is looking for a corresponding change in the training of our doctors. It is no longer feasible for physicians to enter residency or practice without at least a minimal acquaintance with therapies utilized by more than 40 percent of the population. This paper will focus on undergraduate medical education, although postgraduate and continuing medical education in CAM are of equal importance.

* I am well aware that many medical educators and health care professionals object to the term "Complementary and Alternative Medicine", preferring "Integrative Medicine". While I agree that this is a better appellation in many ways, I will for the present continue to use the term used by the National Center for Complementary and Alternative Medicine and the acronym, CAM.

Where Are We Coming From?

In 1996-97, an American Medical Association survey reported 46 schools with CAM as part of a required course.[3] By 1998, 75 of the 125 US medical schools reported offering stand-alone electives, or including CAM topics in required courses.[4] Since that time it is apparent that the interest of the public has continued on an upward trend. The questions is, have medical schools responded to the challenge of preparing doctors who can confidently and helpfully advise a patient who asks about the safety of popular herbal remedies, or the advisability of using acupuncture, ayurvedic medicine, or any one of a dizzying array of potions, nostrums, and palliatives now readily available? Now, more than ever, we need well-trained, knowledge-able physicians who can help patients find their way through the maze of advertising hype, internet information, and conflicting opinions by health care professionals.

There are hopeful signs. During the past few years, the interest of the medical education community has been exhibited by overt action. Examples include the conference at the University of Pennsylvania in November, 1999 entitled "Complementary and Alternative Medicine in the Academic Medical Center: Issues in Ethics and Policy", conferences co-sponsored by the University of California, San Francisco, and Harvard University in November 1998 and May 2000; and the second annual meeting of a consortium of medical schools hosted by the University of Arizona in September, 2000. The Association of American Medical Colleges (AAMC) has co-sponsored conferences on spirituality in medicine with the National Institute for Healthcare Research ((NIHR) and has included issues of spirituality, culture, and end-of-life in their Medical School Objectives report.[5] The CAM Special Interest Group of the AAMC, convened by Patricia Muehsam, MD, of the Mount Sinai School of Medicine, has carried the interest of medical educators forward and painted a vision for the future.[7] Student groups flourish on university campuses including the University of Washington, Brown, Harvard, Johns Hopkins and many others.

Many hospitals now offer a wide variety of alternative and comple-mentary therapies unavailable and unheard of in US hospitals only a few years ago. In Boston, Kathi Kemper, MD, MPH heads the Center for Holistic Pediatric Education and Research at Children's Hospital.[7] The Dana Farber Cancer Institute offers acupuncture, massage therapy, therapeutic touch, herbal/nutritional consultations, and other CAM therapies in conjunction with regular, prescribed medical treatment through their newly-established Leonard P. Zakim Center.[8] Shiatsu, Reiki, aromatherapy and other CAM modalities are available in many hospitals and through some HMOs and managed care organizations.[9] The appointment of Stephen Straus, MD to head the National Center for Complementary and Alternative Medicine (NCCAM) has been hailed as a move that will earn respect from many members of the allopathic medical community.[10] Inevitably, mainstream medicine is making room for CAM in the patient-care arena.[11]

While CAM activity abounds in hospitals, private offices, and specialized CAM clinics, the medical curriculum has been slower to change. We face, first of all, the inertia of huge educational institutions in which most medical schools are embedded. In many cases, any significant change in curriculum requires a long and arduous process. Then, too, advocates of CAM are having a difficult time defining the core knowledge, skills, and attitudes needed by the doctors, nurses, and other health care workers of tomorrow. We are in much the same situation as the proverbial blind men examining the elephant. No consensus exists as to which of the many treatment modalities, philosophical approaches, and belief systems should be included in the well-rounded curriculum.

NCCAM has offered some help by delineating six fields of complementary and alternative medicine:[12]

— Diet, nutrition, lifestyle change, mind-body control;

— Bioelectromagnetic applications;

— Alternative systems of medical practice;

— Manual healing;

— Pharmacological and biological treatments;

— Herbal medicine.

Not surprisingly, these have undergone revision from time to time, and do not represent universal agreement.

A Sampling of CAM Educational Programs

A brief description of undergraduate CAM educational activities in a sampling of US medical schools follows. Nine of the programs described are from schools that sent representatives to the second annual meeting of the Consortium on Integrative Medicine convened at Miraval, Catalina, Arizona, September 8-10, 2000. They represent the breadth and variety of CAM activities in US medical schools at the present time. All have administrative support at the Dean's level. The conference dealt with CAM research, patient care, and medical education from undergraduate to CME. Our focus here is on the four years leading to the MD degree.

Albert Einstein College of Medicine of Yeshiva University

Until 1999, the preclinical integrative medicine curriculum at AECOM consisted of one eight-week elective course and one afternoon workshop in the Introduction to Clinical Medicine course. A standing committee of faculty members, convened by Associate Dean for Educational Affairs, Dr. Albert Kuperman, is currently planning an expanded curriculum that will be integrated into all four years of the existing undergraduate curriculum. The most significant and easily-accessed opportunities for this integration are expected in the present problem-based and case-based learning curricula already in place. A number of cases that include elements of CAM are already under development, and faculty development is planned during the coming year to prepare the discussion group leaders.

The clinical CAM curriculum to date has consisted of fourth year electives offered by the clinical faculty in the affiliated Montefiore and Beth Israel Family Practice programs. These electives provide a one-month opportunity for students to observe the clinical practice of a broad range of CAM modalities including chiropractic, herbal medicine, mind/body approaches, osteopathic manipulation, and acupuncture. These electives can each accommodate only one student per month, and demand far exceeds availability. In addition, students do extensive reading on CAM topics and prepare a research paper applying an evidence-based approach to one discipline or to CAM treatment options for one particular disease entity.

The affiliated Continuum Center for Health and Healing (CCHH) will provide a clinical site to expand the availability of third and fourth year electives, and will serve as the focus for a larger, more comprehensive clinical experience to reinforce the CAM content of the pre-clinical curriculum.[13]

University of Arizona College of Medicine

The University of Arizona is best known for developing the first postgraduate fellowship program in Integrative Medicine. Thus far, the Program in Integrative Medicine (PIM) has had 12 integrative medicine fellows and four pediatric research fellows under the NCCAM Center for Pediatrics grant. In addition, 42 physicians are enrolled in a two-year distributed learning associate fellowship inaugurated in August, 2000.

The University of Arizona's undergraduate medical education includes an elective for first- and second-year students, a fourth-year month-long elective and a resident rotation. Required lectures on integrative medicine are incorporated into the Social and Behavioral Medicine course. The course directors for Preparation for Clinical Medicine and Histology have recently agreed to work with PIM to incorporate integrative medicine materials into their syllabi. Victoria Maizes, MD is the Interim Medical Director of PIM.[14]

Duke University School of Medicine

An innovative pilot course, Complementary Medicine: Academic and Community Perspectives, was taught to a multidisciplinary group of 40 students in the Fall of 1999. It consisted of a series of three-hour joint presentations by Duke faculty and CAM practitioners. In April, 2000, six fourth-year medical students participated in a one-month pilot elective, which consisted of intensive instruction in self-care skills and visits to community CAM practitioners. This course received very high evaluations, with the students strongly recommending that it be shifted into earlier years in the curriculum

A weekly series of noon lectures was initiated in May, 2000 to provide information on herbs to correlate with the material being taught in the first-year Pharmacology course. A follow-up pilot program was initiated for the first calendar block of the 2000-2001 academic year as a required Biochemistry/Nutrition evening case correlation series. Menus for accompanying meals were carefully chosen to correlate with the biochemistry curriculum and supported with patient case presentations and Duke faculty evidence-based presentations on related topics.[13]

Georgetown University School of Medicine

Under the leadership of Aviad Haramati, Ph.D., Georgetown University School of Medicine has embarked on a five-year project of curriculum development in CAM. The broad objective is to develop and implement an educational program that incorporates and integrates CAM information into both the basic science and clinical curriculum so that all students graduating from Georgetown University School of Medicine will have an improved level of awareness of CAM information and practices and will thus be able to communicate more effectively with their patients and provide them with a more comprehensive and integrative approach to health care.

For the past 20 years, students at Georgetown have had access to a variety of course offerings that include CAM information, such as the Mind Body Medicine course in the Department of Psychiatry, taught by Dr. James Gordon, and case-based small group discussions in the Introduction to Health Care, among others. However, in the current year, CAM material will be integrated into first-year basic science courses that are required of all students. For example, in the Gross Anatomy course, a lecture on the "Anatomy of Acupuncture" was presented in context following the presentation of the anatomy of the back and upper limbs. Plans are to include a discussion of the mechanisms of pain relief by acupuncture in the Neurosciences course in the Spring. Also this year, the Human Physiology course will include discussion of the physiological basis for the Relaxation Response (together with a Yoga demonstration) following the traditional presentation of the Physiology of Stress lecture.[15]

Harvard Medical School

Harvard Medical School has offered a one-month elective, Alternative Medicine: Implications for Clinical Practice and Research, since 1993. David Eisenberg, MD and Ted Kaptchuk, OMD, are co-directors. Major topics in the course include homeopathy, chiropractic, macrobiotic diet, botanicals, therapeutic massage, traditional Chinese medicine, vitamins and cancer therapy, acupuncture, guided imagery, energy/psychic healing, and the placebo effect. Students have the opportunity to experience a number of the therapies first-hand. Lectures and demonstrations are given by local providers of these therapies.

Each week of the course is introduced by a case written from actual patient records. The course emphasizes critical reading of the literature and analysis of research methodology. Each case is accompanied by extensive, carefully selected readings. Students are required to write a proposal for a study of a CAM therapy as a final project for the course.

In addition, at Harvard Medical School there is a large-group CAM session for all third year students in the required Patient-Doctor Relationships course. With the recent establishment of a Division for Research and Education in Complementary and Integrative Medical Therapies, there is interest in making CAM information widely accessible throughout the curriculum.[13]

Jefferson Medical College

The CAM educational program at Jefferson Medical College of Thomas Jefferson University has steadily developed since its inception in 1994. It became incorporated into the Center for Integrative Medicine in 1998. At Jefferson, physicians and non-physicians work together to enrich the therapeutic options for the patients.

The educational program in CAM for medical students extends from the first year of medical school to graduate medical education and CME. For first and second-year students there are required one-hour lectures on "A New Medical Model", "Overview of CAM", "Botanical Medicine" in Pharmacology 101, and a two-hour lecture on "Nutritional Medicine". In addition, the following second-year elective seminars, encompassing 15 contact hours, are offered twice a year: Sophomore Seminar on CAM, Sophomore Seminar on Mindfulness-Based Stress Reduction (MBSR), and a new Sophomore Seminar on Medical Yoga. There is a one-hour lecture on "Botanical Medicine" as part of the senior elective, Pharmacology 401, and a four-week course, Senior Clinical Elective in Integrative Medicine. This is a supervised preceptorship experience that allows students to spend time with physician and non-physician providers of complementary therapies. Students complete a course of directed reading and prepare a final paper for presentation.

In a related medical humanities program that is a required segment of a first-year core course, students in small groups spend a structured 3-1/2 hour afternoon at the Philadelphia Museum of Art exploring works of art representative of worldviews that speak to the nature of suffering and healing. There is also a two hour required presentation within the first-year core course, Doctoring in Health and Illness, that utilizes Joseph Campbell's description of the Hero mono-myth to explore the common cycle of separation, initiation, and return traveled by doctors and patients, and an additional lecture this year on the values that underly the Hippocratic tradition.[16]

Mount Sinai School of Medicine of New York University

Three courses are available to the students at Mount Sinai School of Medicine. The first is Integrative Approaches to Health Care. It is a survey course designed to give a broad overview of the field. Topics include Non-allopathic systems (Traditional Chinese Medicine, Ayurveda, Homeopathy, Naturopathy), Biologic and Pharmacologic Approaches, Functional Medicine, Western Botanical Medicine, Manual Therapies, Energetic Therapeutics, Mind-body approaches, and Diet/nutrition/lifestyle approaches.

Class time is divided into one-half didactic presentation and one-half experiential. There are discussions about the nature of science and critical thinking. One class features a panel of patients who talk about their experiences with CAM. The class meets for two hours per week for one semester. Elective credit is given.

The other two courses are clinical electives: Clinical Experiences in Oriental Medicine, and Integrative Approaches to Health in Clinical Practice. In the former students meet with a wide variety of practitioners in the community, and in the latter, students meet with course director Patricia Muehsam, MD and observe her practice which draws from the disciplines of Asian and Western medicine. There is a strong emphasis on self-care, with students learning techniques of meditation, breathing, yoga, and others.[17]

University of California, San Francisco, School of Medicine

The Osher Center for Integrative Medicine, established in 1997, is taking a leading role in the major revision of the UCSF medical school curriculum to be implemented in the Fall of 2001, according to Interim Director, Ellen Hughes, MD. There are plans to design an evidence-based program in integrative medicine that will be integrated into the required curriculum via cases, and to design an extensive web-based curriculum in integrative medicine that will be accessible to the CAM community and the schools of medicine, nursing, pharmacy, dentistry, and physical therapy at UCSF.

Examples of presently existing elective courses are: Mindfulness-Based Stress Reduction Program for Medical Students, Herbal Medicine and Dietary Supplements, the Healer's Art (Rachel Naomi Remen and 11 voluntary faculty teach this popular elective to more than half of the first and second-year medical students), Complementary Paths of Healing (a survey course in CAM), and a "Matching" Program with UCSF medical students and students from local CAM colleges.

New courses to be offered are a month-long fourth-year elective that will focus on critical evaluation of CAM literature and a fourth-year exchange program with the American College of Traditional Chinese Medicine. Other collaborative relationships have been forged with schools of Pharmacy, Nursing, Physical Therapy, and numerous departments within UCSF, and with Harvard University, Kaiser Permanente, Hahnemann College of Homeopathy, and the American College of Traditional Chinese Medicine outside UCSF.[13]

University of Maryland School of Medicine

The Complementary Medicine Program (CMP) at the University of Maryland, under the direction of Brian Berman, MD, includes 16 hours of CAM-focused education in the core curriculum. Lectures are given in the first, second, and third years, along with a student-driven problem-based learning case and two small group sessions in the second year. There is also a CAM elective of approximately 120 hours offered to fourth-year students.

Educational efforts have also been extended to Family Medicine residents, and a CAM Distinguished Speaker Series, featuring lectures by noted academicians in the field of CAM, has been initiated as the first step in the development of a CME program. As part of an NIH P-50 center grant, the CMP is involved with a Career Development Program for junior faculty and fellows. The program offers training and mentorship in research and complementary therapies with the objective of nurturing the next generation of complementary medicine researchers.[18]

University of Minnesota Medical School

Led by the Senior Associate Dean of Education, Greg Vercellotti, MD, and the Director of the Center for Spirituality and Healing, Mary Jo Kreitzer, PhD, RN, the medical school is currently evaluating and strengthening the entire four-year curriculum. A set of competencies have been developed that will permeate the entire four-year curriculum.

Competency I -   Culture, Explanatory Models and Health Care;

Competency II -   Mind-Body-Spirit Relationships;

Competency III - Healing Systems and Practices;

Competency IV - Integrative Medicine Skills

Specific expectations are spelled out for each competency and addressed in required courses including Spirituality (Clinical Medicine I, II, IV); Cultural Dynamics (Clinical Medicine I); and Herbal Medicine (Pharmacology). Additional integrative medicine topics woven throughout the required curriculum include: Diverse Healing Therapies (TCM, Chiropractic, naturopathic care), Legal, Ethical, and Health System Issues, Intra- and Inter-professional Challenges, and Self-awareness and Self-care. Elective opportunities in years III and IV include a three-week experiential seminar in Complementary and Alternative Medicine, and a preparatory course for international clinical experience.

The Center for Spirituality and Healing is also noted for offering the nation's first interdisciplinary graduate minor in complementary therapies and healing practices.[19]

University of Pennsylvania School of Medicine

During the past few years, the medical center has explored the role of CAM in its academic mission of education, research and clinical practice. As part of a major revision of the medical curriculum that began in 1997, CAM (regarded as a complementary rather than alternative therapy) has been increasingly incorporated into the teaching of medical students. This process has been guided by Alfred P. Fishman, MD, Senior Associate Dean for Program Development and Chair of the Steering Committee on Complementary Therapies at Penn working with Gail Morrison, MD, Vice-Dean for Education. Instead of focussing on lectures, emphasis has been placed on strategic introduction of CAM modalities into relevant components of the medical curriculum so as to raise students' awareness of unconventional therapies, to inform them about how consumers may be using these therapies and to alert the students about possible interactions of herbs and medications and of adverse reactions.

Introduction of CAM into the medical curriculum has benefited greatly from prior implementation of a successful nutrition education program at Penn. For example, relevant aspects of herbal medicine have become part of conventional instruction on cardiovascular disease, gastrointestinal disease and reproduction. Instruction in CAM is planned to extend beyond the campus to the medical school's "virtual curriculum" on the Internet.

In introducing CAM, advantage has been taken of the themes of professionalism and the patient-doctor relationship, which permeate the medical curriculum. For example, since 1998, the "Doctoring Course", which runs through the four-year continuum, has included seminars on CAM and stress management. In addition to the structured curriculum of required courses, electives are available for hands-on experience with expert practitioners during the clinical years. Moreover, evening courses, open to the medical community as well as students, offer lectures on diverse topics, ranging from alternative systems, such as Ayurveda and Chinese Medicine, to individual complementary therapies, such as Yoga and Massage. These courses have been well attended by students, house staff and faculty.

Finally, student interest in CAM has let to the formation of a student Alternative Medicine Interest Group that is supported by the University and sponsors seminars and evening symposia.

Trends

Several trends are apparent in these brief descriptions, and in discussion with medical educators interested in helping CAM find its rightful place in the medical curriculum. First, there is a strong trend toward incorporating and including CAM topics in the core curriculum, rather than adding stand-alone courses. If future physicians are to integrate these therapies into their way of approaching clinical care, they must acquire knowledge of their use at the same time they are developing their basic medical knowledge and skills. Inclusion alongside what are commonly regarded as the basic medical sciences will help the student to see the equal value of the art and science of medicine, and to recognize the necessity of both in the care of the patient. This is not to imply that we should discard the excellent elective CAM courses that have been developed at many medical schools. Learning theory tells us that actual experience is a powerful means of learning.[20] CAM rotations or courses over an extended period of weeks are often able to incorporate a strong experiential component that cannot be included elsewhere.

A second trend, tentatively beginning, is the idea of cross-training between allopathic and CAM schools (see UCSF). Not only do patients want physicians who are knowledgeable about CAM; a growing number of medical students, residents, and physicians in practice also recognize the need to acquire CAM knowledge and skills. These opportunities have been available at the graduate level,[21, 22] but have rarely been offered to undergraduate medical students. The problem of a place in the curriculum will have to be resolved, but exchange rotations for students in allopathic medical schools and students in chiropractic, naturopathic, homeopathic, and other CAM schools would seem to be mutually enlightening.

Another benefit of cross-training is to enhance team building. Working in teams is now an essential skill in many endeavors, especially in health care. Few patients are cared for by one health professional. The majority of people who see CAM practitioners also see a primary care provider, or one or more medical specialists. A recent Josiah Macy, Jr. Foundation-sponsored conference was convened to study ways to enhance interactions between nurses and doctors. They concluded that this is important first of all for the benefit of the patient.[23] The same principle applies to CAM and allopathic physicians working together. All parties, including the patient should be on the same team.

Most CAM courses in allopathic medical schools are not expected to teach CAM skills to a level of clinical competence. Rather, they are designed to give the student an understanding of the therapy, its uses and possible effects. There are already an unknown number of medical doctors who are also fully trained in acupuncture, chiropractic, homeopathy, and any number of CAM therapies, and who practice an eclectic type of medicine, utilizing all of their skills. One might confidently predict that this number will increase in response to patient demand and the physician's desire to be competent in a broader range of therapies.

A third trend is the inclusion of the concept of self-care for the student and future physician in the medical curriculum. There is a growing realization that many of the traditions of medical training (sleep deprivation; poor nutrition; and lack of time for exercise, meditation, and recreation) are detrimental to health and establish poor habits that may last a lifetime. Furthermore, they represent hypocritical behavior, in that physicians advise their patients to do otherwise.[24] To change this situation will require serious re-thinking of present medical education practices and policy, especially in the clinical years. The trend toward health maintenance and disease prevention rather than an exclusive focus on disease treatment will make it more evident that physicians should be role models for their patients.

Needs

As these trends emerge, several needs that we have known about all along become more apparent. The first is the need for sound science in support of CAM therapies.[25, 26] With increased grant support from the National Center for Complementary and Alternative Medicine there is more research under way than we could have imagined a few years ago. Grants of 8 million dollars each to Johns Hopkins University and the University of Pennsylvania were recently announced by NCCAM, bringing the number of funded Centers studying the underlying mechanisms and health effects of CAM therapies to fifteen.[27] While we await the results of these studies with interest, we should remain open to the possibility that our present ways of doing research may not provide all of the answers when dealing with complementary and alternative therapies. In spite of our advances in medical science, there is still a great deal we do not fully understand about the functioning of the human body, mind, and spirit. This is an exciting frontier for our present medical students, and all the more reason we should teach them to think critically and innovatively.

As mentioned previously, the field of CAM needs to arrive at some general consensus about the essentials of a core curriculum. Not that there ever could or should be complete unanimity, but that there be some agreement on areas that all medical students should master. This could be based on the classification scheme developed by NCCAM, or on a taxonomy of what physicians should know to be able to advise patients about 1) therapies that are proven efficacious; 2) therapies that are probably harmless; and 3) therapies that are potentially dangerous. There should be sound instruction about the very real dangers of drug/herbal interactions, and issues about harmful delay of conventional treatment. Of equal importance, and previously lacking in the training of doctors, is a knowledge of the concomitant use of conventional treatment and alternative therapies when conventional medicine has failed to bring about improvement, or for palliation in serious or painful illness.

While consensual thinking would bring some structure to the vast and diverse field of CAM education, medical school faculties and curriculum planners should carefully consider what they want their own students to know and be able to do when they graduate, taking into account their own unique institutional culture, resources, and values.

Finally, there is always the need for a valid assessment system for student achievement and program evaluation. This is the educational conundrum that is often inadequately addressed and never fully resolved. Perhaps even more than in other areas of medical education, the usual testing of facts will not suffice in CAM. A better understanding of learning theory[20] can help us to design assessments that are meaningful and worth the time spent on them by both faculty and students. If we are expecting administrative and financial support for CAM in the medical curriculum, we may be sure that we will be asked to produce some evidence that resources are well-spent. Observational assessments such as the Observed Structured Clinical Examination (OSCE) are widely used and accepted. If we include CAM components in the curriculum, we should expect to observe students asking questions about the use of herbs and other CAM therapies in the patient interview, and demonstrating an expected level of competence by including them in treatment plans.

Future Directions

There is no doubt that we are in the midst of major changes in health care. Many of these changes are putting added stress on health care providers and patients alike. We wonder how we can find the time, money, and energy to cope with these changes. At the same time, CAM can be a positive influence. We recognize the wisdom of our bodies in maintaining health, and the wisdom of the ages in health practices of all people. CAM has been a major influence in turning our thinking from curing disease to promoting health.

It will continue to help us look beyond the bounds of conventional thinking to find new ways of understanding. Our task now is to keep the momentum moving in a positive direction.

A follow-up survey of educational activities in CAM is now underway. It is hoped that the resulting information can be updated on a regular basis and made readily available to everyone who is interested.

References

1. Eisenberg D.M., Kessler R.C., Foster C., Norlock F.E., Calkins D.R., Delbanco T.L. Unconventional medicine in the United States: prevalence, costs, and patterns of use. *NEMJ*, 1993;328:246-252.

2. Eisenberg D.M., Davis R.B., Ettner S.L., Appel S., Wilkey S., VanRompay M., Kessler R.C. Trends in alternative medicine use in the United States, 1990-1997: Results of a follow-up national survey. *JAMA*, 1998;280:1569-1575.

3. American Medical Association Council on Medical Education. Encouraging medical student education in complementary health care practices. Chicago, IL: American Medical Association, June 1997.

4. Wetzel M.S., Eisenberg D.M., Kaptchuk T.J. Courses involving complementary and alternative medicine at US medical schools. *JAMA*, 1998;280:784-787.

5. Association of American Medical Colleges. *Reporter*, 1999;9(2), Cohen J.J. Learning to listen, p. 2; "Neglected" skills headline latest *MSOP* report, p. 5.

6. Muehsam P.A. Alternative and complementary medicine annual meeting activities. *GEA Correspondent.* Spring, 2000:8.

7. Integrated Medicine Alliance newsletter, March, 2000. Boston, MA.

8. Dana Farber Cancer Institute. Impact, 2000:3(1), and Leonard P. Zakim Center information packet.

9. Pelletier K.R., Astin J.A., Haskell W.L. Current trends in the integration and reimbursement of complementary and alternative medicine by managed care organizatons (MCOs) and insurance providers: 1998 update and cohort analysis. *American Journal of Health Promottion*, 1999 14(2):125-133.

10. Stokstad E. Stephen Straus's impossible job. *Science*, 2000;288:1568-1573.

11. Marshall E. Bastions of tradition adapt to alternative medicine. *Science*, 2000; 288:1571-1572.

12. National Center for Complementary and Alternative Medicine (NCCAM) website: http://nccam.nih.gov/nccam, 2/1/2000.

13. Adapted from information provided for the program syllabus of the Consortium on Integrative Medicine, Miraval, Catalina, Arizona, September 8-10, 2000.

14. Information supplied by Victoria Maizes, M.D., Interim Medical Director, Program in Integrative Medicine, University of Arizona College of Medicine.

15. Information supplied by Aviad Haramati, Ph.D., Education Project Leader, Georgetown University School of Medicine.

16. Information supplied by Steven Rosenzweig, M.D., Director, Center for Integrative Medicine, Jefferson Medical College at Thomas Jefferson University.

17. Information supplied by Patricia A. Muehsam, M.D., Course Director, Mount Sinai School of Medicine of New York Univesity.

18. Information supplied by Brian Berman, M.D., Director, Complementary Medicine Program, University of Maryland School of Medicine.

19. Information supplied by Mary Jo Kreitzer, Ph.D., R.N., Director, Center for Spirituality and Healing, University of Minnesota Medical School.

20. Coles C. How students learn: the process of learning. In Jolly B, Rees L., eds. Medical Education in the Millennium. New York: Oxford University Press, 1998.

21. Kemper K.J., Vincent E.C., Scadapane J.N.. Teaching an integrated approach to complementary, alternative, and mainstream therapies for children: A curriculum evaluation. *Journal of Alternate and Complementary Medicine* 1999;5(3):261-268.

22. Cummings M, Lemon M. Combined allopathic and osteopathic GME programs: A good thing, but will they continue? *Acad Med* 1999;74(9):948-950.

23. Ryan S. Enhancing Interactions Between Nursing and Medicine: Opportunities in Health Professional Education. Chairman's summary of conference to identify ways to strengthen the professional relationship between medicine and nursing, sponsored by the Josiah Macy, Jr. Foundation, July 2000.

24. Hatem C.J.. Physician, heal thyself. Harvard Medical Alumni Bulletin, Summer, 2000: 16-19.

25. Devries J.M. Emerging educational needs of an emerging discipline. *Journal of Alternate and Complementary Medicine* 1999;74(9):269-271.

26. Jobst K.A., Murphy D.G. Alternative medicine, education and standards of publication and research. *Journal of Alternate and Complementary Medicine* 1999;74 (9):221-222.

27. NCCAM announcement on Intelihealth Professional Network web site, www.Intelihealth.com, 10/6/00.

A Taxonomy of Complementary and Alternative Medicine

Marc S. Micozzi, M.D., Ph.D.
College of Physicians of Philadelphia

The public's expectations of physicians have never been higher than they are today. As we enter the 21st century, the patient's agenda includes the expectations that physicians and other health providers will be knowledgeable and able to offer helpful advice about what we call complementary and alternative medicine.

The fact is that our patients have already voted. It is estimated that as many as 50 percent of American adults now use one or more complementary therapies on a regular basis. In many cases, they do so knowing that there may be no third-party payer willing to pick up the cost, so it represents the last bastion for traditional fee-for-service medicine. The *Wall Street Journal* reported several years ago that Americans were already spending 20 billion dollars a year on complementary medical approaches. Viewed from another perspective, it is estimated that there are more annual patient visits to alternative providers than to primary care physicians.

As you know, trust is a fundamental foundation of the doctor-patient relationship. For years, many patients were either too embarrassed or simply unwilling to tell their primary care physicians about their use or visits to complementary health providers. This is the very situation that every conscientious physician wants to avoid. Fortunately, available research indicates that this situation is changing. Now when patients come to us with questions or concerns about complementary medical approaches, we'll be able to give useful answers to them.

Complementary or Alternative Therapies

A semantic observation is in order. The word "alternative," or the term "alternative medicine," seems to be culturally encoded in the English language to encompass a wide spectrum of systems, styles, techniques, and modalities of health care. It has also developed an exclusionary connotation. It is not that there are many alternatives to biomedicine but that biomedicine is one of many alternatives.

Many who work in the field prefer to use the term "complementary medicine," which has been used in the UK. This is a more accurate description of the social phenomenon in the United States because patients in this country use "alternative medicine" as an adjunct to, and not primarily a replacement for, conventional medical care. Much of what we call complementary medicine in the US represents time-honored traditions of medical practice originating from other countries and other cultures, or from the history of health practices in European and American society itself.

One of the most important distinctions we should make is to note the differences between two types of practices. The first are those that are many years or centuries old and have a large body of practitioners and patients and a well-developed fund of clinical "wisdom" that is encoded into the belief system of a particular society or subgroup of people. But a separate category lumped into alternative medicine includes practices that have been developed more recently by one or several practitioners in isolation from peers and without benefit of scientific testing and clinical study, what I sometimes call "unusual therapies and practices". Practices in that category often fit conceptually within the biomedical model but simply have not been tested by use of the standards of biomedical research and practice.

Medical Belief Systems

Those who work in medicine and health care typically refer to "the art and science of medicine." We do so, in part, because patients and physicians alike come to the treatment process with expectations of various kinds, and those expectations are shaped largely by cultural considerations. Americans may belong to different HMOs, or none at all, but each of us does belong to a medical belief system about health and healing, just as people in other nations have cultural medical systems of their own.

Speaking in general terms, a medical belief system is a complex of beliefs, models, and linked activities that providers and users consider useful in bettering health and well-being, and in relieving stress and disease. The components of such a system include:

— A developed theory of the body/person known as the explanatory model. This theory includes the causes and malfunction as well as appropriate ways to address this malfunction;

— Plans to educate and train new practitioners through apprenticeship or schooling;

— A health care sub-system that delivers care to the needy;

— Associated means of producing substances or technologies necessary to deliver care;

— Professional organizations of practitioners who monitor each others' practices and promote the system to potential users;

— A legal mandate that provides for the official recognition of practitioners and maintains the minimum standard of quality; and

— A social mandate that informally reveals levels of community acceptance by frequency of use, willingness to pay, and stereotypes about practitioners, among other markers.

Biomedical Complexity of Health Systems

This lengthy definition makes it clear that a health care system is complex and multi-layered, and that there is a hierarchy of scale in the resort to medical therapies. Even simple systems, such as those limited in scope to one self-defined ethnic group, may be difficult for one person to wholly master or describe. Larger systems are correspondingly more complex, encompassing a wide range of viewpoints, numerous sub-specialties and distinctive styles of practice.

Biomedicine includes specialties ranging from the intensely material practice of surgery to the far more relational specialties of family medicine and psychiatry. Biomedical complexity is compounded by the fact that it is practiced differently in different countries.

Even the best simultaneous translator may have trouble dealing with the fact that peptic ulcer and bronchitis do not mean the same things in Britain as they do in the US, that the US appendectomy becomes the British appendicetomy and that the French tendency to exaggerate means that there are never headaches in France, only migraines, and that the French often refer to real migraines as "liver crises". The German language has no word for chest pain, forcing the German patient to speak of heart pain. When a German doctor says cardiac insufficiency, it may simply mean that the patient is tired. How can biomedicine, which is commonly supposed to be a science, be so different in four countries where people relatively share a similar cultural background? The answer is that while biomedicine benefits from a base of scientific input, culture intervenes at every step of the way.

This complexity is equally true of Chinese medicine, which embraces many styles including traditional Chinese medicine, Five Element Style, Japanese, Korean, and French style. Even community-based or folk systems may have different specialties. The Lakota or Sioux people distinguish medicine men and women who emphasize herbal treatment from holy men and women who practice shamanically. The Navajo recognize three types of diagnosticians and singers who work with rituals, herbs and the psychological body to deliver health care.

Individual Practitioners in the Complex Health System

So, health systems are a product of a culture's world view. Very much smaller scale in the system is the style of technique or therapy in terms of a style an individual practitioner uses and the techniques he or she employs reflect the system. A technique is comparatively simple. It may be a single therapy and often can be practiced without being linked to an explanatory model, without detailed training or without professional oversight. Some practitioners specialize in offering single therapies such as bee sting injections, colonic irrigations, biofeedback, specific dietary supplements or Swedish massage.

Single therapy practitioners can provide symptomatic relief to their patients, but they cannot provide systematic care, that is care guided by a well-developed model of how the body person works, how the malfunction arose, and how the technique can help. Indeed, the expanse of power and persistence of health care systems correlate with the effectiveness of their explanatory models and linked therapeutic modalities.

Explanatory Models of Health Care Systems

Where do these models come from? As noted earlier, health care systems are embedded in the sociocultural systems surrounding them. This provides not only access to natural resources but also to ideas, assumptions and patterns of logic. All these are reflected in the explanatory models and health care delivery formats and health care ideas that society can encompass.

Nevertheless, certain world views tend to predominate in the world today. In the United States and Europe, the hierarchic or reductionist world view dominates. This world view model emphasizes hierarchies of value, a tendency to be judgmental, competition, forcefulness and materialism. Biomedicine reflects these patterns in its concern for the expertise of the practitioner and its tendency to magnify the importance of some specialties or diseases over others, such as cardiac surgery or cardiology over pediatrics and cancer over asthma. Its preferences for treatment modalities caused obvious reactions to the physical body, and its focus on endstage physical malfunction to paying less attention to less developed conditions and rejecting non-material explanations of cause.

Cartesian assumptions permeate western society and form the *modus operandi* of conventional medicine. They have led the belief in rationalism, causality, objectivity and, for example, the separation between (bio)medicine and psychiatry. The assumptions work very well in acute emergency situations, but are more limited when illnesses become chronic. In Chinese cosmology, Cartesian thinking may be classified broadly as "yang" and its inferred opposite is "yin." Chinese philosophic thought can therefore be seen to be inclusive of Western thought while Western thought does not easily incorporate Chinese holistic thinking.

Some Western health belief systems originated in reaction to biomedicine, which was called myelopathy by the homeopaths in 1842, and those systems that responded in reaction to allopathic medicine include homeopathy, osteopathy, and naturopathy as well as chiropractic and Christian Science in American history. Others have been imported from Asia: Chinese medicine and Ayurveda from India. All of these other systems argue, not always convincingly, that their approaches to care are more egalitarian, less judgmental and gentler than biomedicine. Some offer non-materialistic explanations of cause and cure, and in making such arguments call upon another world view currently held in the United States, mainly the relational, ecological or holistic world view.

This world view sees all things as connected in the network of relationships and deals with how people, things and energy interact, and how these interactions can better the whole. Reflected in health care, this idea means that practitioners model health in terms of achieving balance and patients are seen to have expertise also different from that of the practitioner but expertise nonetheless. Thus practitioner and patient form a partnership and patients take responsibility for their own care and development.

Current Complementary/Alternative Therapies in the United States

I would like to offer some definitions of the most significant complementary approaches in this country today:

Homeopathy is a method of self-healing thought to be assisted with small doses of medicinal substances and practiced by licensed physicians and other healthcare practitioners throughout the world. In the US, homeopathic medicines are regulated by Federal law and most are over-the-counter.

The homeopathic method was developed by Samuel Hahnemann, a German physician, chemist, and author of a well-known textbook on the preparation and use of contemporary medicines who lived from 1755 to 1843. In a series of experiments, from 1790 to 1810, Hahnemann demonstrated that medicinal substances elicit a standard array of signs and symptoms in healthy people and the medicine whose symptom picture most closely resembles the illness treated is the one most likely to initiate a curative response from the patient. Hahnemann took these experiments to mean that the outward manifestations of illness represent the concerted attempt of the organism to heal itself and that the corresponding remedy reinforces that attempt in some way. He coined the term homeopathy to describe his method of using remedies with the power to resonate with the illness as a whole, in contrast to the conventional method of opposing symptoms with superior force.

Homeopathy does not place patients into diagnostic pathologic categories, but is focused on description and alleviation of symptoms through an empirical process of "provings." Since this process involves a great deal of listening to and talking to the patient, with its own proven therapeutic benefits, and since many symptoms improve by themselves, a homeopathic proving is not tantamount to a clinical trial.

Chiropractic was born in the American Midwest a century ago. This manual healing art has matured to mainstream status while preserving its essential tenets. The modern profession has become part of the health care establishment with licensure, an increasingly strong scientific research base, widespread insurance coverage, and approximately 20 million patient visits per year in the US, while maintaining strong roots in the alternate health community with a philosophy that emphasizes healing without drugs. Spinal manipulation has been documented for millennia and both Hippocrates and Galen were advocates of this technique.

During the second half of the 19th century, the US became a vibrant center of natural healing theory and practice. During this time, osteopathy, developed by Andrew Taylor Still, evolved as another manual based healing art. Daniel David Palmer, a self-educated healer, in the Mississippi river town of Davenport, Iowa, founded the chiropractic profession in 1895 on two fundamental principles: that vertebral subluxation (a spinal misalignment thought to cause abnormal nerve transmission) is the cause of virtually all disease; and that chiropractic adjustment (a manual manipulation of the subluxated vertebra) is it's cure.

This "one cause-one cure" philosophy played a central role in chiropractic history. While few if any contemporary chiropractors will endorse this simplistic formulation, it remains true that the *raison d'etre* of the profession is the detection and correction of spinal subluxation. Chiropractors do more, but it is their ability to do this one thing that has allowed their art to survive for a century until recently under constant medical opposition.

Healing touch is one of a long line of healing traditions based on the belief in the universal healing of energy and is a contemporary American manifestation of ancient traditions perhaps best called "energy healing." As one of these energetic healing strategies, healing touch includes new techniques as well as modern variations of indigenous practices found around the world. Energetic strategies are credited with relieving physical and emotional distress. Some approaches use a practitioner's hands to interact with a person's energy flow.

Early references to universal energy are found in India as early as 5000 B.C. Since then, many cultures have developed rich philosophies in healing traditions around this concept. Some terms used to describe this phenomenon are prana in India, ch'I, qi, and ki in China, Thailand, and Japan, and mana in Polynesia. A common, contemporary energetic healing approach is the Krieger-Kunz technique of therapeutic touch. This is seen as a type of pranic healing, a modern interpretation of several healing practices that may collectively be called the "laying on of hands".

Other practices that were transplanted to Western society are reflexology, raki, and acupuncture, and naturopathy, or naturopathic medicine, which grew out of alternative healing systems of the 18th and 19th centuries but traces its philosophic roots to the Hippocratic school of medicine. Over the centuries, natural medicine and biomedicine have alternatively diverged and converged, shaping each other, often in reaction to each other. The term naturopathy was coined in 1895 by John Scheel of New York as he described his natural methods of health care. But early forerunners of these concepts already existed in the history of natural healing, both in America and the Austro-Germanic European core.

Naturopathy became a formal profession due to the ethic of Benedict Lust, a German immigrant, who came to the US in 1892 when he was 23. Lust defined naturopathy as "nature-cure", both a way of life and a concept of healing that employed various natural means of treating human infirmities and disease states. The earliest therapies associated with the term involve the combination of American hygienics and Austro-Germanic nature-cure and hydrotherapy. Today, because of the conscious intent of naturopathic medicine to bring any and all modalities to bear on healing the patient, I sometimes refer to naturopathic medicine as "neo-eclectic" medicine.

Ayurveda is the best known of the traditional approaches associated with Indian medicine. The reliance in Ayurveda on the three doshas as explanations for cause and as means for cure can be likened to constitutional medicine and the Sheldon somatotypes of physical anthropology. The idea that physical constitutions are related to disease is currently found in biomedicine with our investigation of molecular genetics and the promise of genetic therapy. Dissection of the human genome may be seen as yielding to the ultimate units of human anatomy. So, the idea that constitution relates to disease is something we pursue in biomedicine by other means.

The history of Indian medicine occurred in four main phases. The first, or Vedic phase dates from about 1200 to 800 B.C. Information about medicine during this period is obtained from numerous incantations and references to healing that are found in the *AtharVaveda* and the *Rigveda*, two religious scriptures that describe a magical, religious approach to healing. In fact, these two Vedas provide the classical antecedents to the current practice of yoga.

The second, or classical, phase is marked by the advent of the first Sanskrit medical treatises, the Caraka and Sushruta Samhitas, which probably date from a few centuries B.C. to several centuries A.D. This period includes subsequent medical treatises dating from before the Muslim invasions of India in the beginning of the 11th century, for these works tend to follow the earlier classical guidelines and provide a basis of traditional Ayurveda.

The third, or syncretic, phase is marked by clear influences on classical Ayurveda from Islamic or Unani, south Indian Sissha, and other nonclassical medical systems. Bhavamishra's 16th century Bhavaprakahia reveals the results of these influences, which included diagnosis by examination of pulse or urine. That phase extends from the Muslim influences to the present era which encompasses "Maharishi Ayurveda," which I think of as "New Age" Ayurveda or the classic paradigm revisited and adapted to the world of science and technology including relations to quantum physics, mind/body science, as well as advanced biomedical science. This recent manifestation of Maharishi Ayurveda, although most visible in the Western world and perhaps something that was designed with the Western world in mind, is actually slowly filtering back into India itself.

Traditional Chinese Medicine

We can think of the traditional medicine of China as an empirical tradition of systematic correspondences making reference to five cosmic elements, going back to roughly 3000 B.C. Although for comparative purposes Chinese medicine is often treated as a homogenous or monolithic structure, this view neglects the changing interpretations of basic paradigms offered by Chinese medicine through the ages and synchronic plurality at any point in time, with differing opinions and ideas over thousands of years. Some scholars have described Chinese medicine as a system that never threw anything away.

Much of what the Chinese medical practitioner does is thought to influence the flow or balance of the body's energy, called qi. In my view, the Chinese concept of qi which is translated as energy, bioenergy or vital energy, has a metabolic quality because the Chinese character for qi may be described as vapor or steam rising over rice. The term rice has a specific quality that we associate with a specific food, but it also has a generic meaning "food" or foodstuff. For example, the character "rice hall" is used to describe a restaurant in Chinese. The elusive meaning of qi may therefore be likened more to living metabolism than to the energy that we associate with electromagnetic radiation.

But energy, or qi, also has the dynamic qualities of flow and balance. Because flow and balance are dynamic, they could be described in changing terms from one patient to the next or in the same patient from one day to the next, again not using static or fixed pathologic diagnostic criteria. Such concepts represent great challenges in translation to the biomedical map.

<u>Acupuncture</u> is a major modality for the manipulation of qi and even though we think of the fine filiform needle that we are familiar today, Chinese practice through history has had all kinds of different instruments for influencing qi. Clinical observations of the efficacy of acupuncture are increasing and some biomedical explanations focus on the physiologic effects of skin puncture and/or modulation of neurotransmitter substances. Other experiments have more to do with the flow of energy itself.

Mind Body Healing

As we look across this history and heritage of health and healing, it is clear that health is not about a given medical system or tradition. It is about the mind and the body and how they work and how they can heal. Formulary approaches — that is techniques taken out of their health care systems or traditions such as formulary acupuncture, formulary herbalism, formulary homeopathy — are still seen to sometimes have effects on the body. It may be that these formulary approaches, taken out of context and providing clinical efficacy, give evidence that empirical traditions may have discovered truths about human physiology and encoded them into culture belief systems.

Nonetheless, no medicine works well if the patient or the practitioner does not believe in it, and any medicine works better if both patient and practitioner believe in its efficacy. The health care practitioner operates in and between the realms of art and the science of medicine. Integration of complementary and alternative medicine into medical practice affords the opportunity to expand our knowledge of both.

Section II

Complementary Medicine in the Academic Health Center

Evidence, Ethics, and the Evaluation of Global Medicine

Wayne B. Jonas, M.D., Uniformed Services of the Health Sciences, and Klaus Linde, M.D., Technical University, München, Germany

Introduction

Complementary and alternative medicine (CAM) is a set of medical practices that is not part of conventional care but still used by patients in their health care management. These practices have increased in popularity in recent years, emerging as an area of great public interest and activity, both nationally and globally.[1] The current definition of CAM creates a category of health care and medical practices that is wide and variable, ranging from nutritional and behavioral interventions to ancient and comprehensive systems such as ayurvedic and traditional Chinese medicine. As the use of CAM practices rises, obtaining reliable information about the safety, effectiveness and mechanisms of these practices requires rigorous investigation. This paper discusses issues important for evaluating these practices.

Conventional physicians often refer to others for CAM and, to a lesser extent, provide CAM services. In a review of 25 surveys of conventional physician referral and use of CAM in the United States, Astin found that 43 percent of physicians referred patients for acupuncture, 40 percent for chiropractic and 21 percent for massage.[1] The majority believed in the efficacy of these three practices. Use of CAM practices by physicians was much lower ranging from 9 percent (homeopathy) to 19 percent (chiropractic and massage).[2] Organizations such as the British and American Medical Associations and the Federation of State Medical Boards in the United States have called on physicians to learn about CAM, discuss these practices with their patients, and incorporate them into proper clinical management.[3,4]

The Potential Risks and Benefits of CAM

Many CAM practices, such as acupuncture, chiropractic manipulation, homeopathy, and meditation, are low risk but still need to be used by competently trained practitioners in order to avoid misuse.[3] Some CAM practices, such as acupuncture, require extensive training and skill to deliver properly, yet, conventional physicians are legally allowed to use such practices even if they may not have received adequate training or certification in in their use. The adequacy of

118

training of CAM practitioners also varies — many having no certification or state licensing and overview procedures at all.

Herbal preparations are readily available over-the-counter and contain powerful pharmacological substances, which can be toxic and produce herb-drug interactions.[5] These herb-drug interactions may be quite significant and hard to detect without concerted basic and clinical investigation. For example, St. John's Wort, an herb considered quite safe and commonly used for the treatment of depression and dysthymia has recently been reported to accelerate drug metabolism of antiretroviral and cytotoxic agents resulting in increased viral load in HIV infected patients and organ rejection in transplant patients.[6, 7] Herbs need the same phase I and II clinical testing as pharmaceuticals to assess pharmacodynamics and drug-herb interactions before moving into large scale clinical trials or marketing. This testing is complicated by the fact that many herbs have multiple or unknown active ingredients making such testing difficult. Thus, systematic post-marketing surveillance is especially important. Adulteration, contamination, and poor quality control are also possibilities with these products, especially if shipped from Asia.[8] Safety monitoring and product quality seem to be the minimum evidence necessary for marketing. Evaluation of efficacy with large randomized trials is difficult in herbalism due to the modest effect sizes, paucity of funding, and their use primarily in chronic, non-life-threatening conditions.

Some CAM practices have clear value for the treatment and prevention of disease. In botanical medicine, for example, there is research showing benefit of herbal products such as *ginkgo biloba* for improving multi-infarct dementia[9] and possibly Alzheimer's;[10] benign prostatic hypertrophy with saw palmetto and other herbal preparations;[11, 12] and the prevention of heart disease with garlic.[13, 14] It appears that St. John's Wort is effective in the treatment of depression and produces less side effects and costs less than some conventional antidepressants.[15] The quality of many of these trials is poor, however, with small sample sizes, variable outcome measures and lengths of follow-up and differing product standards.

The Scientific Method in Medicine

Clinical research in CAM needs the same rigorous research methods developed for conventional medicine. Sometimes more rigor is required because of the complexities and implausibility of CAM practices. There are six types of research frequently used in the investigation of medicine and the type of information these approaches provide varies. These include:

1. **Qualitative research methods**. This includes detailed case studies and patient interviews that describe diagnostic and treatment approaches and investigate patient preferences and relevance. Qualitative approaches have been developed in anthropology and are becoming increasingly common in nursing and primary care.

2. **Laboratory and basic science approaches**. These methods investigate the basic mechanisms and biological plausibility of medical practices. *In vitro* (cell culture, intra-cellular such as with probe technology) and *in vivo* (testing in normal, disease prone or genetically altered animals) are now extensively used and expanding into molecular realms.

3. **Observational studies.** These methods include practice audit and epidemiological research, outcomes research, surveys and other types of observational research. These studies may not have a comparison group or they may attempt to create comparison groups by sampling patients not treated with the intervention.

4. **Randomized controlled trials (RCTs)**. This method attempts to isolate the specific contribution of different interventions on selected outcomes. Such studies usually involve the assignment of patients to one treatment group or another using a random method. Various approaches are used to make group assignments such   as randomly selected numbers or computer-generated random assignment. The best approach involves concealing knowledge of which patients will get which treatment at the time of assignment (allocation concealment).

5. **Meta-analysis, systematic reviews**. These approaches and less rigorous approaches such as expert review and evaluation are methods for assessing the accuracy and precision of clinical research. Criteria-based systematic reviews are increasingly being used in place of subjective reviews.

6. **Health technology assessment and health services research**. These are a collection of approaches for examining the utility and impact of interventions in the light of treatment delivery factors such as access, feasibility, costs, practitioner competence, patient compliance, etc. This may take the form of surveys or sampling from groups already getting an intervention to evaluating quality of care, costs and other factors. Random sampling may or may not be used.

Differential Goals of Research Types

Certain groups may preferentially seek out one or more of these research methods and the type of information they provide. For example, basic scientists may have more interest in the results of laboratory research, clinicians more interest in the results of clinical trials, etc. Laboratory research, randomized controlled trials and systematic reviews or meta-analyses are testing for the existence of a specific effect from an intervention or are used to support a theory about mechanisms. Qualitative research, observational trials or health technology assessment are testing for the probability, magnitude and relevance of an effect in clinical practices or health care delivery systems. There may be tension between research that tries to isolate specific effects (laboratory, RCTs, meta-analyses, etc.), and research that tries to define the utility, public impact and relevance of a practice in the real world (qualitative, observational and health services, etc.). Since one can rarely address more than one question in a single research project designing research that attempts to address both specific and pragmatic questions simultaneously is problematic. To address both specificity and utility, carefully developed research and evaluation strategies are needed to prevent each method from being interpreted in isolation. Consistent decision rules for the evaluation of research is an important step in the continued development of science-based medicine.[16] To understand the relationship between different types of research methods, we must be able to judge the quality of research on the basis of its goals.[17]

Quality Criteria for Research on CAM

Evaluation of complementary and alternative medicine is fundamentally no different from evaluating conventional medicine.[18, 19] There are, however, certain conceptual and contextual issues of which investigators should be aware when evaluating research on CAM topics.[20] The validity of randomized controlled trials, for example, involves a set of quality criteria that test "internal validity" or the likelihood that observed effects are biased. The applicability of information from clinical research, including RCTs and observational trials, criteria for "external validity" or the likelihood that the observed effects will occur in varied situations are used. The Consolidated Standards of Reporting Trials (CONSORT) group has produced a widely adopted set of reporting guidelines for RCTs.[21, 22] These guidelines emphasize the importance of allocation concealment, randomization method, blinding, proper statistical methods, attention to drops-out and other factors.[23, 24]

Model Validity

In addition to internal and external validity, research on CAM requires additional criteria that address "model validity", or the likelihood that the research has adequately addressed the diagnostic taxonomy and therapeutic context of the CAM system.[25] Many complementary medicine practices come from systems of therapeutics developed outside these standard assumptions of western medicine. Therefore, it is important to consider the interaction of research methods with the conceptual systems being investigated. For example, some CAM treatments are investigated in populations for which the practice is integral to the culture and may produce variation in responses even when standardized.[26] Individual expectations within a culture and the nature of the information given to patients (including the informed consent procedure) can also impact outcomes significantly.[27, 28] "Model validity" in the evaluation of CAM research involves addressing these factors.

Diagnostic Taxonomy

In a clinical trial, an investigator first collects a "homogeneous" group of patients with a common diagnosis. When this "homogenous" group is evaluated from the perspective of another medical tradition, however, these patients may not be homogenous. Research not incorporating these variations in patient classification can be problematic.

For example, a homogenous group of osteoarthritis patients from the western perspective may represent over a dozen treatment groups when evaluated by traditional Chinese medicine (TCM). A "standardized" treatment can approximate the "average" syndrome and is the way many investigators handle this situation. Standardization has advantages in that it simplifies the treatment strategy, may allow for blinding and may prevent treatment confounding. It has the disadvantage of providing suboptimal treatment and so may produce "false negative" results. That is a problem of model validity. For example, Bensoussan conducted a study of patients with irritable bowel syndrome.[8] One third of the patients were treated with individualized traditional Chinese medicine, one third were treated with a standardized Chinese medicine approach and one third served as controls, receiving placebo. Subjects treated with the TCM model improved for longer than those given the standardized approach. Both groups did better than the placebo control group.[29]

Double Classification

Another approach to the different diagnostic taxonomies in alternative medical systems is that of double classification and selection in clinical trials. Initial selection criteria are made according to standard Western medicine then additional criteria are applied according to the alternative system. This double classification approach is possible in many situations but adds considerable complexity to the study and increases the likelihood that the trial will produce ambiguous results. For example, Shipley conducted a placebo-controlled trial of the homeopathic remedy *Rhus toxicum* on a "homogenous" group of osteoarthritis patients without careful classification according to the homeopathic "model" and reported no effect of *Rhus toxicum* over placebo.[30] Fisher, in a follow-up investigation, used a "double selection" approach for testing *Rhus toxicum* that provided both good internal validity and model validity. Patients had to meet strict criteria for fibromyalgia and *Rhus toxicum* producing a group of subjects "homogenous" for both systems of medicine. In this study patients treated with homeopathy did better than those given placebo.[31] Such studies are more complicated and may require more resources than the average drug study.

Adequacy of Treatment

A standardized approach can lead to inadequate treatment. For example, in a study of acupuncture of HIV-associated peripheral neuropathy a "standardized" approach to treatment was used. To do this, the investigators had to markedly alter what most TCM acupuncturists do in such cases. The study reported the results as negative, yet many acupuncturists report good results when using TCM principles in this condition.[32] Considerable time, collaboration and testing are needed in order to work out the best balance between internal, external and model validity factors when evaluating CAM. How to determine when adequate treatment has occurred may not be simple. For example, acupuncture is more like physical therapy or surgery than drug therapy and is applied in very different ways with different skills. If one treatment style is interpreted as *the* acupuncture treatment, it must be optimal or at least *representative*, for a defined group of providers. This has implications for the design and strategy of acupuncture research. For example, in a review of 15 randomized trials of acupuncture for asthma we found very different treatment approaches.[33] Only two trials used the same acupuncture points, and these were by the same author.

Placebo and Non-specific Effects.

The observed benefits of many alternative medical practices are often attributed to "placebo" or "non-specific" effects. It is not unusual to see 70-80 percent effectiveness from many practices both conventional and alternative.[34, 35] Traditional Chinese medicine, ayurveda, Native American medicine and various mind/body and spiritual healing approaches induce self-healing partly by manipulating the context, meaning and interpretation of illness and outcomes. Manipulation of "meaning" (the placebo aspect of treatment) can interact with specific therapies in complex ways.[26, 27, 36] Many traditional medical practices provide sophisticated ways of producing these "meaning effects." Arthur Kleinman's classic studies of why traditional healers provide relief illustrated the importance of contextual issues for all medicine.[37] The interaction of these specific and contextual or "placebo" effects is an important area for focused research.[38]

Smoking cessation is of particular interest in regard to the placebo problem and some CAM therapies. For example, research on smoking cessation shows that there is clear evidence that acupuncture acts like "placebo" acupuncture.[39, 40] While there is no difference in smoking cessation rates between acupuncture and "placebo" acupuncture — there is also no difference between acupuncture and proven effective smoking cessation treatments.[40] Thus, acupuncture, in spite of being a placebo, appears to be equally effective as a conventional intervention! How can we deal with this paradox? The rationale that we are simply fooling patients with placebo is too simplistic an interpretation to be useful. Certainly an important part of the solution is to ask patients if they care if they stop smoking because of a "placebo" effect or a "specific" effect by an otherwise safe and inexpensive procedure.

The introduction of placebo controls and blinding enhances and confuses the conclusions of clinical research in acupuncture. What is an adequate placebo control for acupuncture? Should we use stimulation of non-acupuncture points, or points thought not to be indicated, or superficial needling, or the use of devices using ultra-sound, electrical or laser stimulation, which are switched off for the placebo condition? Deep needling techniques are unlikely to be inert. Procedures without needling are likely to be distinguishable. The question that matters most to patients (and most physicians) is not its specific effects but whether acupuncture benefits patients. Patient-oriented acupuncture research would include careful, multi-dimensional measurement of outcomes, inclusion of independent (and if possible, blinded) evaluators and rigorous monitoring. This type of research approach might be better for many conditions than the use of questionable placebo controls.

Selecting Patient or Theory Relevant Outcomes and Designs

An outcome that is easy to measure may be substituted for or used to represent other outcomes that may be more important for patients or groups of patients. Cassel and others have pointed out that may occur because an overemphasis on trying to find a "cure" may distract us from healing illness, one of the core goals of medicine.[41] This occurs when there is an overemphasis on conducting efficacy studies that maximize "internal validity" using objective measures at the expense of "external" and "model" validity. Selection of outcomes that are irrelevant to patients is more likely to occur when researchers select the study outcome without adequate patient input. For example, Cassidy did interviews with over 400 patients who visited acupuncturists and explored the reported benefits.[42, 43] Most patients did not have major improvement of their western diagnosis, however, they continued to return for acupuncture treatment because of an improved ability to "manage" their illness and a sense of well-being after acupuncture. This type of outcome is not easy to measure "objectively" in clinical trials and so is rarely incorporated into research design. Clinical researchers investigating CAM need to pay special attention to selecting outcomes that address the most important patient concerns for their illness. This may require adding a person and process (such as qualitative research methods) for identifying such outcomes when designing the trial.

Finding the balance between rigorous *evidence* and patient *relevance* is illustrated with two examples from acupuncture. Because of its simplicity, more than 30 trials have investigated P6 acupuncture in the study of nausea and vomiting with positive results.[44] It is a simple intervention, easily standardized, and also studies a condition where outcomes are straightforward and follow-up is short. It is the most studied area in acupuncture largely because it is easy to study. The findings are not very useful for the acupuncturist, however, who rarely uses only P6 when treating this condition. More important to the public than nausea are conditions such as chronic pain, stroke rehabilitation and drug addiction where placebo-controlled evidence is much less convincing;[45, 46] but these are more difficult to study in independently repeated rigorous clinical trials.

A similar dilemma exists when evaluating homeopathy, another CAM system in which research has narrowly focused on the placebo question. However, placebo in clinical trials of homeopathy has different meaning than in conventional medicine. For example, if a specific chemical is tested in a placebo-controlled trial there is usually no question about its biological activity regardless of its clinical usefulness. Homeopathic remedies in high dilutions, however, are usually assumed, *a priori*, to be inactive. Thus, clinical trials in homeopathy are only partly "true" clinical trials in a conventional sense. This is because they try simultaneously to answer the question of clinical efficacy and also what would usually be considered a basic science question addressed in laboratory research. Mixing those questions into a single trial is not a reasonable strategy, since it produces ambiguous answers to both questions. Not only do these studies not answer the placebo questions, they are largely irrelevant for improving the practice of homeopathy. The most investigated clinical models in homeopathy are of *Galphimia glauca* for hay fever,[47] Opium, Raphanus, Arnica or China for postoperative ileus (see ref. 48 for review), and homeopathic immunotherapy for allergic rhinitis.[49] The remedy Galphimia and the homeopathic immunotherapy approach are rarely used by homeopaths. To use either alone would be considered a suboptimal application of the therapy. Likewise, postoperative ileus is hardly ever treated with homeopathy. As in acupuncture, these conditions have been studied because they are easy to study, not because they are relevant to patients or practice. The pressure to answer the question of placebo with rigor in all clinical research can result in neglect of research most relevant for practice. In addition, it also fails to answer the placebo question.[48]

Hypothesis Testing

Hypothesis-generated research is the method by which we identify cause and effect relationships in medicine. It is a powerful method for studying and confirming pre-identified therapy-outcome links. A drawback of hypothesis-generated research is that by focusing on *a priori* theoretical associations that explore particular theory-driven outcome links, we run the risk of establishing prematurely, conclusions about the ultimate value of a therapy, and we also restrict exploration of other, possibly better, therapies.[50] Once treatments are established using hypotheses generated from a single perspective they become "standard of care," and alternative treatments are then more difficult to explore. For example, coronary artery by-pass grafting (CABG) is an established treatment of coronary artery disease (CAD). This treatment assumes an anatomically based hypotheses about the etiology of CAD. An extensive industry has developed around this procedure. Lifestyle therapy can also treat CAD but is based on a non-anatomical hypothesis of CAD etiology. Lifestyle therapy might be superior to CABG in the treatment of CAD given its low cost, preventive potential, reduction in fatigue and improvement in wellbeing.[51-54] However, adequate comparison of lifestyle therapy vs. CABG is problematic largely because perceptions and resources are already committed to CABG. We do not know if either hypothesis about the etiology of CAD is correct because neither approach can be tested in placebo-controlled trials. In the early 1960s sham surgery of internal mammary ligation produced positive effect rates similar to what CABG produces today.[55] Sham testing cannot be done for CABG today even though the contribution from placebo effects in surgery may be large.[56, 57] Thus, hypothesis formation and testing in clinical research can be a double-edged sword by revealing partial causes and yet running the risk of obscuring more fundamental knowledge and exploring more beneficial therapies for chronic disease. Clinical research for disease with complex and multi-factorial causes should provide for research strategies that test multiple hypotheses.[58-60]

The Value of Randomization

Randomization has value in science and medicine for many, but not all, interventions. In some clinical situations, randomization may assist in revealing true effect sizes. In other cases, for example, in behavioral medicine, it may obscure or have no effect on outcome.[61] Some alternative systems assume that randomization can interfere with important aspects of the therapy and obscure awareness of how bias is occurring. For example, traditional Chinese medicine is based on an assumption that "correspondences" occur across system levels (biological, social, cosmic, etc.).[62, 63] These traditional medical systems view extensive efforts to establish precisely the causal links of an intervention and outcome <u>within</u> a level (as done in RCTs) to be less valuable than is assumed in western medicine.[64]

In some CAM systems practitioner and investigator intent is assumed to have influences on outcomes and experimental results. They assume that the effects of intent are inherent at all levels of the therapeutic and experimental process and can alter and even create apparent chance phenomena.[65] If these assumptions are correct the interaction of bias and randomization is more complex than medical science and statistics currently assume.[66, 67] The extent to which investigator intent is relevant to medical research is unknown. These issues are probably only significant when contradictory information from high quality trials arises. Thus, examining the influence of intentionality can only be done with rigorous research methods and cannot be evaluated if the quality of research is poor. Unfortunately, the quality of research in CAM is rarely that good.[68]

Blinding/Masking and Expectancy Control

While we currently have no completely acceptable way to check for successful blinding, it is still considered an important criterion of quality in research design.[21] Many alternative treatments such as herbal therapies and acupuncture can be blinded, or at least partially blinded. In herbal studies care must be taken to match smell and taste. In acupuncture, usually the practitioner cannot be blinded; whereas in homeopathy a study is easily double blinded. Studies of complex behavioral and lifestyle programs will find blinding impossible. In these cases, however, control for time and attention and blinding of the outcome assessment and analysis is possible. For example, in trials of therapeutic touch, providing equal time for relaxation, a sham therapist can be incorporated into the study design.[69] Blinding the evaluation is accomplished by having an individual or group separate from the therapists do the outcome measurements. Analysis can be done blind by having results coded in a way that does not reveal the intervention to the statistician.

Equipoise and Patient/Practitioner Preferences

Patient and practitioner beliefs also have important consequences for clinical research, especially in CAM. Randomization can be ethically done only when there is true equipoise between treatment groups, that is, when the question of efficacy is truly ambiguous and there is no strong belief about the value of the therapy. Equipoise is usually present when new drugs are tested. This situation rarely exists in alternative medicine, however. Most patients and therapists have been using or avoiding CAM therapies because of strong preferences.[70] This makes recruitment problematic. Several clinical trials of CAM have been stopped either because conventional practitioners would not refer patients to a CAM study or because patients refused to be randomized to the conventional control group.[71] It is known that randomization schemes have been subverted by well-meaning health care practitioners in conventional medicine, a problem that may be even more extensive in trails on CAM.[72] In addition, clinical research may be significantly contaminated when subjects are using other alternative therapies that interact with the treatments being tested. For example, over 16 percent of patients enrolled in clinical trials at the NIH Clinical Center are using herbal therapies. This herbal use is usually not reported to investigators.[73] Patient and practitioner preferences must be carefully considered when designing and managing clinical research on CAM.

Summarizing Research

We live in the information age. Keeping up with the literature even in a small subspecialty is a daunting task. There are currently at least 80 major databases and over 400 journals publishing alternative medical literature around the world. It is not surprising that various research summaries may come to markedly different conclusions. Contributing to differences in interpretation of the literature are publication bias, incomplete access to the literature, poor quality original research, varying standards of evaluation, inaccuracies and disagreements when applying evaluation criteria, failure to use consistent research goals and objectives when selecting and evaluating studies, and differing beliefs about CAM in general.[24, 74, 75] State-of-the-art review methods, such as those developed by the Cochrane Collaboration, should be used, as they provide the best current approach to clinical research summary.[76] Other methods, such as those used to establish practice guidelines, or the NIH Consensus Conference approaches, are usually less systematic and less rigorous for evaluating clinical research.

Risk Stratification and the Level of Scientific Proof

Many therapies, both conventional and alternative, become accepted before convincing evidence from randomized trials is collected.[77] Acupuncture provides a current example of this in CAM. Even in the absence of proof of acupuncture's effectiveness for most conditions for which it is used, positive experiences by patients and an increasing number of physicians are contributing to a growing acceptance of acupuncture in general. The safety of acupuncture made the NIH acupuncture consensus panel willing to recommend it with less evidence than other interventions with a higher risk. Thus, risk stratification (see article by B. Strom in this section) may be a good initial step before deciding on the kind of evidence required for acceptance in CAM. Risk stratification is a key element to balancing rigor and relevance when evaluating research strategies and practicing evidence-based medicine.[78] While more and better randomized clinical trials are clearly important there are a number of preconditions for such trials. These include:

— The investigated treatment should be representative of actual practice for a defined group of practitioners. Representativeness should be demonstrated empirically in observational and outcomes studies. An alternative is to use treatment approaches and qualification standards officially recommended by professional societies.

— Pilot studies are mandatory before starting randomized trials.

— The use of placebo-controlled conditions as a requirement for determining what is adopted in practice is questionable.

— Clinical studies comparing CAM to, or in addition to, standard therapies of proven effectiveness should be used more often. For example, a direct comparison of acupuncture to standard therapy or as an addition to standard therapy is useful if we believe that acupuncture might produce fewer side effects than standard therapy alone, or might reduce cost with equal efficacy.

There is a need for observational studies before extensive, broadly based, controlled trial research is conducted. Practice audit and outcome studies may identify areas of strength and weakness in these practices and so help guide both practice and research.[71]

Matching Goals and Methods in Clinical Research

A recurrent theme in research is the importance of defining clearly the questions being asked, the goals those questions seek to fulfill, and then applying the appropriate methods used to answer those questions.[79] As indicated, there are many types of research methods, each with its own purpose, value and limitations. The quality of these methods should not be judged in isolation, but rather in relationship to the research goals and questions being explored. The decision to pursue a particular approach depends on a number of factors including:

— the simplicity or complexity of the condition and therapy being investigated;

— the type of information sought (causal, descriptive, associative, etc.);

— the purpose for which a particular audience will use the information; and,

— the methods of investigation that are available, ethical and affordable.

For example, a physician considering a patient referral for acupuncture might want to know what kinds of patients the local acupuncturists see, how they are treated, whether patients are satisfied with treatment, and outcomes. This type of information comes from practice audit (observational or outcomes research). Thus, observational designs may be of more value than relying on the results of small-scale, placebo-controlled trials done in another country with practitioners and populations quite different from those in the community. Observational studies must be as performed as rigorously as experimental studies. For CAM theories and data that do not fit into our current assumptions about the nature of reality (e.g. prayer, "energy" healing, homeopathy, etc.) a multi-domain and carefully thought out research strategy is needed. Given the public interest in and the implications for science of these areas it is irresponsible for the scientific community to ignore them completely.[25]

General guidelines for matching goals and methods are as follows:

1. When defining problems and definitions of terms, and when assessing the relevance of outcome measures across diverse

populations, qualitative methods with in-depth interviews and content analysis are necessary.

2. When assessing the incidence, prevalence and associations of variables, the most useful approaches are surveys or cross-sectional and longitudinal studies with methods for construct development and factor analysis.

3. When the goal is to identify the comprehensive impact of complex interventions delivered in the clinical context, pragmatic trials and outcomes approaches should be applied.

4. When attempting to isolate specific effects of treatment on selected outcomes, randomized controlled trials are the method of choice.

5. When exploring mechanisms of action or attempting to determine optimal timing, dosage and combinations for use in clinical trials, laboratory research is needed.

An important part of research evaluation is checking to see that the questions asked and the methods selected are appropriate for each other.[71] Of course, once selected each method must be executed in a rigorous manner.

Assuring Research Quality

For each of the evidence domains, criteria for scientific rigor should be defined in relationship to the particular goals pursued. A number of quality criteria have been described in this chapter. These methods cannot function in isolation, nor do they always stand in a particular fixed hierarchy as is often suggested.[80, 81] Both experimental and observational designs are needed to explore the validity and value of CAM practices and assumptions. Interdisciplinary research involving experts in both conventional and CAM fields are needed. For example the field of psychoneuroimmunology arose because psychologists and immunologists began to conduct collaborative projects bringing together their laboratory and clinical research expertise. Development of other interdisciplinary fields is likely if scientists design projects that cut across research domains without violating quality criteria within each domain. Such exploration would allow us to develop a scientific basis for therapeutic diversity in chronic disease management.

Rigor, Relevance and Realism

Evaluating the safety, effectiveness and mechanisms of CAM practices is complex, and a handful of large-scale randomized trials will not answer even the main questions needed. The resources required for extensive, systematic, cross-domain research will not be available in the next several years even for the most prevalent interventions. Yet, the use of CAM continues to increase. Given this situation, we cannot afford to fix *a priori* on a single research method but must balance our research strategies between a) relevance, b) scientific rigor, and c) feasibility. In addition, studies should address the interests of different audiences that research serves. As a minimum, input on research priorities should be balanced with the interests of 1) patients, 2) providers, 3) the scientific community, and 4) policy makers. Those groups are each interested in overlapping types of information but they may have differing priorities. That will determine different types of research approaches and strategies.

CAM and the Evolution of the Scientific Method

In the past, the interaction of conventional and unconventional medicine has resulted in improvements in the scientific method. For example fifty years ago, methods of blinding and randomization became accepted into orthodox medical research only after they were first applied to unorthodox practices such as mesmerism, psychic healing and homeopathy.[82] Today traditional and cross-cultural medicine challenges us to make explicit the meaning of quality in biomedical science and to show the evidence upon which those quality criteria are based. Thus research in CAM may help us develop decision rules for improving research rigor and for developing a better strategic approach for science in the age of global medicine.

References

1. Eisenberg D.M., Davis R.B., Ettner S., et al. Trends in alternative medicine use in the United States 1990-1997: results of a follow-up national survey. *JAMA*. 1998;280:1569-1575.

2. Astin J.A., Marie A.M., Pelletier K.R., Hansen E., Haskell W.L.. A review of the incorporation of complementary and alternative medicine by mainstream physcians. *Arch Int Med*. 1998;158:2303-2310.

3. Federation of State Medical Boards. Report on Heatlh Care Fraud from the Special Committee on Health Care Fraud. Austin, Texas: Federation of State Medical Boards of the United States, Inc.; 1997.

4. British Medical Association. Complementary Medicine New Approaches to Good Practice. Oxford: Oxford University Press; 1993:5-148.

5. De Smet PAGM, Keller K., Hänsel R., Chandler R.F.. Adverse Effects of Herbal Drugs. Heidelberg: Springer-Verlag; 1997.

6. Ruschitzka F., Meier P., Turina M.. Acute heart transplant rejection due to St. John's Wort. *Lancet.* 2000;355:548-9.

7. Piscitelli S., Burstein A., Chaitt D.. Indinavir concentrations and St. John's wort. *Lancet.* 2000;355:547-8.

8. Bensoussan A, Myers S.P.. Towards a Safer Choice. Victoria, Australia. University of Western Sydney Macarthur; 1996.

9. Kleijnen J, Knipschild P. Gingko biloba for cerebral insufficiency. *Br J Clin Pharm.* 1992;34:352-358.

10. Le Bars P.L., Katz M.M., Berman N., Itil T.M., Freedman A.M., Schatzberg A.F.. A placebo-controlled, double-blind, randomized trial of an extract of ginkgo biloba for dementia. *JAMA.* 1997;278:1327-1332.

11. Di Silverio F., Flammia G.P., Sciarra A., et al. Plant extracts in BPH. *Minerva Urologica e Nefrologica.* 1993;45:143-49.

12. Wilt T.J., Ishani A., Stark G., MacDonald M.S., Lau J., Mulrow C.. Saw palmetto extracts for treatment of benign prostatic hyperplasia. *JAMA.* 1998;280:1604-1609.

13. Neil A., Silagy C.. Garlic: its cardio-protective properties. *Current Opinion in Lipidology.* 1994;5:6-10.

14. Jepson R., Kleijnen J., Leng G.. Garlic for peripheral arterial occlusive disease. *The Cochrane Review.* 1999.

15. Linde K., Ramirez G., Mulrow C.D., Pauls A., Weidenhammer W., Melchart D. St John's wort for depression—an overview and meta-analysis of randomized clinical trials [see comments]. *BMJ.* 1996;313:253-8.

16. Eddy D.M.. Clinical decision making: from theory to practice: a collection of essays from JAMA. Boston: Jones & Bartlett Publishers; 1996:5.

17. Jonas W.B.. Evaluating unconventional medical practices. *Journal of NIH Research.* 1993;5:64-7.

18. Levin J.S., Glass T.A., Kushi L.H., Schuck J.R., Steele L., Jonas W.B.. Quantitative methods in research on complementary and alternative medicine. A methodological manifesto. NIH Office of Alternative Medicine. *Med. Care.* 1997;35:1079-94.

19. Vickers A., Cassileth B., Ernst E., *et al.* How Should We Research Unconventional Therapies? *International Journal of Technology Assessment in Health Care.* 1997;13:111-121.

20. Eskinaski D.P.. Factors that shape alternative medicine. *JAMA.* 1998;280:1621-1623.

21. Begg C., Cho M., Eastwood S., et al. Improving the quality of reporting of random-ized controlled trials. *JAMA.* 1996;276:637-639.

22. Moher D. CONSORT: an evolving tool to help improve the quality of reports of ran-domized controlled trials. *JAMA.* 1998;279:1489-1491.

23. Stroup D.F., Berlin J.A., Morton S.C., et al. Meta-analysis of observational studies in epidemiology. *JAMA.* 2000;283:2008-2012.

24. Egger M, Davey S.G., Altman D.G.. Systematic Reviews in Health Care: Meta-analysis in Context. London: BMJ Books; 2000.

25. Jonas W.B.. Researching alternative medicine. *Nature Medicine.* 1997;3:824-827.

26. Moerman D.E.. Cultural variations in the placebo effect: ulcers, anxiety, and blood pressure. *Medical Anthropology Quarterly.* 2000;14:51-72.

27. Bergmann J., Chassany O., Gandiol J., Deblois P., Kanis J., *et al.* A randomized clinical trial of the effect of informed consent on the analgesic activity of placebo and naproxen in cancer pain. Clinical Trials and Meta-Analysis. 1994;29:41-47.

28. Kirsch I.. How Expectancies Shape Experience. Washington, DC: American Psychological Assoc; 1999.

29. Bensoussan A., Talley N.J., Hing M., Menzies R., Guo A., Ngu M.. Treatment of irritable bowel syndrome with Chinese herbal medicine. *JAMA.* 1998;280:1585-1589.

30. Shipley M., Berry H., Broster G., Jenkins M., Clover A., Williams I. Controlled trial of homeopathic treatment of osteoarthritis. *Lancet.* 1983;i:97-98.

31. Fisher P., Greenwood A., Huskisson E.C., Turner P., Belon P. Effect of homeopathic treatment on fibrositis (primary fibromyalgia). *Br Med J.* 1989;299:365-366.

32. Shlay J.C., Chaloner K., Max M.B., *et al.* Acupuncture and amitriptyline for pain due to HIV-related peripheral neuropathy. *JAMA.* 1998;280:1590-1595.

33. Linde K., Worku F., Stör W., *et al.* Randomized clinical trials of acupuncture for asthma - a systematic review. *Forsch Komplementärmed.* 1996;3:148-155.

34. Jonas W.B.. Therapeutic labeling and the 80 percent rule. *Bridges.* 1994;5:1, 4-6.

35. Roberts A.H., Kewman D.G., Mercier L., Hovell M.. The power of nonspecific effects in healing: implications for psychological and biological treatments. *Clinical Psychology Review.* 1993;13:375-91.

36. de Craen A.J., Moerman D.E.. Gastrointestingal diseases and their treatment with placebo. In: Moerman D.E., ed. OAM/NIH Conference on Placebo and Nocebo Effects: Developing a Research Agenda. Bethesda, MD: National Institutes of Health; 1996.

37. Kleinman A.,. Eisenberg L., Good B.. Culture, illness, and care: clinical lessons from anthropologic and cross-cultural research. *Ann Intern Med.* 1978;88:251-8.

38. Moerman D., Jonas W.B.. Toward a research agenda on placebo. *Advances in Mind-Body Medicine.* 2000;16:33-46.

39. White A., Resch K., Ernst E.. Smoking cessation with acupuncture? A best evidence synthesis. *Forsch Komplementarmed.* 1997;4:102-105.

40. White A., Rampes H.. Acupuncture in smoking cessation. In: Lancaster T., Silagy C., eds. Tobacco addiction module of The Cochrane Database of Systematic Reviews. Oxford. The Cochrane Collaboration: Update Software; 1997.

41. Cassel E.. The nature of suffering and the goals of medicine. *NEJM.* 1982;306:639-645.

42. Cassidy C.M.. Chinese medicine users in the United States, Part I: utilization, satisfaction, medical plurality. *J Altern Complement Med.* 1998;4:17-27.

43. Cassidy C.M.. Chinese medicine users in the United States, Part II: preferred aspects of care. *J Altern Complement Med.* 1998;4:189-202.

44. Vickers A.J.. Can acupuncture have specific effects on health? A systematic review of acupuncture antiemesis trials. *J Royal Soc Med.* 1996;89:303-11.

45. ter Riet G., Kleijnen J., Knipschild P. Acupuncture and chronic pain: a criteria-based meta-analysis. *J Clin Epidemiol.* 1990;43:1191-1199.

46. ter Riet G., Kleijnen J., Knipschild P. A meta-analysis of studies into the effect of acupuncture in addiction. *Br J Gen Pract.* 1990;40:379-382.

47. Wiesenauer M., Ludtke R.. A meta-analysis of the homeopathic treatment of polynosis with *Galphimia galuca. Forschende Komplenemtarmedizin.* 1996;3:230-234.

48. Linde K., Clausius N., Ramirez G., et al. Are the clinical effects of homeopathy all placebo effects? A meta-analysis of randomized, placebo controlled trials. *Lancet.* 1997;350:834-843.

49. Taylor M.A., Reilly D., Llewellyn-Jones R.H., McSharry C., Aitchison T.C.. Randomized controlled trial of homoeopathy versus placebo in perennial allergic rhinitis with overview of four trial series. *Brit Med J.* 2000;321:471-476.

50. Heron J.. Critique of conventional research methodology. *Comp Med Res.* 1986;1:10-22.

51. Blumenthal J.A., Levenson R.M.. Behavioral approaches to secondary prevention of coronary heart disease. *Circulation.* 1987;76:1130-7.

52. Ornish D., Scherwitz L.W., Billings J.H., *et al.* Intensive lifestyle changes for reversal of coronary heart disease. *JAMA.* 1998;280:2001-2007.

53. McDougall J.. Rapid reduction of serum cholesterol and blood pressure by a twelve-day, very low fat, strictly vegetarian diet. *J of the American College of Nutrition.* 1995;14:491-496.

54. Haskell W.L., Alderman E.L., Fair J.M., et al. Effects of intensive multiple risk factor reduction on coronary atherosclerosis and clinical cardiac events in men and women with coronary artery disease. The Stanford Coronary Risk Intervention Project (SCRIP). *Circulation.* 1994;89:975-90.

55. Cobb L.A., Thomas G.I., Dillard D.H., Merendino K.A., Bruce R.A.. An evaluation of internal-mammary-artery ligation by a double-blind technic. *N Engl J Med.* 1959;260:1115—1118.

56. Beecher H.K.. Surgery as placebo. *JAMA*

57. Johnson A.G.. Surgery as placebo. *Lancet.* 1994;344:1140-2.

58. Gallagher R., Appenzeller T. Beyond reductionism. *Science.* 1999;284.

59. Coffey D.. Self-organization, complexity, and chaos: the new biology for medicine. *Nature Medicine.* 1998;4:882-885.

60. Horwitz R.I.. Complexity and contradiction in clinical trial research. *Am J Med.* 1987;82:498-510.

61. Lipsey M.W., Wilson D.B.. The efficacy of psychological, educational, and behavioral treatment: confirmation from meta-analysis. *American Psychologist.* 1993;48:1181-1209.

62. Porkert M. The Theoretical Foundations of Chinese Medicine - Systems of Correspondence. Cambridge: The MIT Press; 1974:368.

63. Unshuld PU. Medicine in China. A History of Ideas. Berkeley: Univ of California Press; 1985.

64. Lao L. Traditional Chinese Medicine. In: Jonas W.B., Levin J.S., eds. Essentials of Complementary and Alternative Medicine. Philadelphia, PA: Lipincott Williams & Wilkins; 1999:216-232.

65. Dossey L. Reinventing Medicine: Beyond Mind-Body to a New Era of Healing. New York, NY: Harper San Francisco; 1999:271.

66. Radin D.I., Nelson R.D., Evidence for consciousness-related anomalies in random physical systems. *Foundations of Physics.* 1989;19:1499-1514.

67. Jahn R.G. Consciousness, information and health. *Alternative Therapies.* 1996;2:32-38.

68. Linde K., Jonas W.B., Melchart D, Willich S. The methodological quality of randomized controlled trials of homeopathy, herbal medicines and acupuncture. *International Journal of Epidemiology.* 2001; (in press).

69. Gordon A. The effects of therapeutic touch on patients with osteoarthritis of the knee. *Journal of Family Practice.* 1998;47:271-277.

70. Furnham A., Kirkcaldy B. The health beliefs and behaviours of orthodox and complementary medicine clients. *British Journal of Clinical Psychology.* 1996; 35:49-61.

71. Linde K., Jonas W.B. Evaluating complementary and alternative medicine: the balance of rigor and relevance. In: Jonas W.B., Levin J.S., eds. Essentials of Complementary and Alternative Medicine. Philadelphia, PA: Lipincott Williams & Wilkins; 1999:57-71.

72. Schulz K.F., Chalmers I., Hayes R.J., Altman D.G. Empirical evidence of bias. *JAMA.* 1995;273:408-412.

73. Sparber A., Johnson E., Derenzo E., Bergerson S., Jonas W., White J. Biomedical research and patient utilization of natural herbal products: a case study. *Cancer Investigation.* 2000;18:436-439.

74. Oxman A.D., Guyatt G.H. Guidelines for reading literature reviews. *Canadian Medical Association Journal.* 1988;138:697-703.

75. Angell M., Kassirer J.P. Alternative medicine: the risks of untested and unregulated remedies. *NEJM.* 1998;339:839-841.

76. Bero L., Rennie D. The Cochrane Collaboration. *JAMA.* 1995;274:1935-1938.

77. Eddy D.M. Should we change the rules for evaluating medical technologies. In: Gelijns A.C., ed. Modern Methods of Clinical Investigation. Washington, D.C.: National Academy Press; 1990 :117-34.

78. Jonas W.B., Linde K., Walach H. How to practice evidence-based complementary and alternative medicine. In: Jonas W.B., Levin J.S., eds. Essentials of Complementary and Alterantive Medicine. Philadelphia: Lippincott Williams & Wilkins; 1999.

79. Feinstein A.R. Models, methods and goals. *Journal of Clinical Epidemiology.* 1989; 42: 301-308.

80. Sackett D.L., Haynes R.B., Guyatt G.H., Tugwell P. Clinical Epidemiology: A Basic Science for Clinical Medicine. Boston: Little, Brown, & Co.; 1991.

81. Fontanarosa P.B., Lundberg G.D. Alternative medicine meets science. *JAMA.* 1998; 280:1618-1619.

82. Kaptchuk T.J., Intentional ignorance: the history of blind assessment and placebo controls in medicine. *Bull Hist Med.* 1998;72:389-433.

The Complementary Medicine Program

Brian Berman, M.D.*
Director, Complementary Medicine Program
University of Maryland School of Medicine

The University of Maryland Complementary Medicine Program was founded in 1991 by Brian Berman, M.D. A family practitioner trained at the University of Maryland, Dr. Berman traveled widely to learn about approaches to healing that were unfamiliar to western-trained physicians. After qualifying as a fellow of the faculty of homeopathy in Great Britain and being awarded a diploma in traditional Chinese medicine, he integrated these therapies into his clinic in London for eight years. His awareness of the benefit to patients of an approach that offered greater health care choices and more emphasis on self-care was matched by a simultaneous frustration at the lack of scientific evidence to validate this alternative approach. Without more scientific basis to support the effectiveness and safety of these approaches, the medical establishment would be unwilling to accept it and CAM would remain on the fringe of health care. Thanks to a $1 million grant from the Laing Foundation of Great Britain, matched with resources and funding from the University of Maryland School of Medicine, Dr. Berman was able to return to the US and establish a comprehensive program of research, education and integrated clinical care in CAM.

The administration of the School of Medicine and the hospital would best be characterized, at the time, as embracing an attitude of healthy skepticism; they were open to allowing the project to happen as long as it did not claim to "have all the answers" and was willing to pursue a strong scientific agenda. The program began as a project called, "The Integration of Complementary and Orthodox Medicine," within the University of Maryland Pain Clinic, expanding the clinic to be multi-disciplinary, integrating both conventional and CAM approaches. Fortunately, the private foundation support provided seed funding for a program of pilot studies to be embarked upon immediately. These studies were crucial in generating preliminary data that allowed the program to be competitive in applications to funding institutions such as the NIH. The program now has a large research base with NIH-funded pre-clinical and clinical trials as well as an NIH Specialized Research Center grant in complementary medicine.

* The following is a synopsis of a longer presentation made by Dr. Berman at the meeting.

The structure of the program has changed over the ten years of its existence as it has grown and expanded in all its activities. In 1995 the School of Medicine has created a full Division of Complementary Medicine within the Department of Family Medicine, giving the program greater autonomy and control of its budget while also giving it the scope to function within a primary care discipline. The present structure, created in 1998, is that of an inter-departmental "program" (the highest University status before becoming a full department) within the school of Medicine. In this capacity the program collaborates with, and serves as a resource for, other departments and schools in the University as well as other research institutions nationally and internationally. The program has a staff of 35 including 11 faculty members who get their academic appointments through the Department of Family Medicine. The program director reports to the Dean. Overall support of the program comes through NIH-funded research, private foundation grants and the School of Medicine.

The program's research agenda was created based on surveys of CAM therapy usage rates, conditions identified as major public health problems, and review of the existing CAM literature. As a result of this process the program has focused on pain-related conditions and has initially examined therapies where there was the greatest body of evidence suggesting their usefulness, as well as evidence of their use by consumers. This approach has also led to a diverse and fruitful array of collaborations from the Departments of Rheumatology, medicine and Epidemiology to the Dental School.

At the heart of the program is its integrative medical clinic, the Center for Healing. It is from here that the inspiration for all the work stems – the care of patients. Perhaps the most important added bonuses of the clinic include the excellent opportunity it affords to build bridges with medical colleagues through shared patient care, and its role in generating ideas for collaborative research endeavors. There have been some interesting instances where some of the most skeptical research collaborators have resorted to acupuncture for relief of their own pain conditions. Personal experience of relief has often done more to change attitudes than objective research data! Obstacles the clinical program has faced include distrust and unfamiliarity with CAM therapies being offered under the University's umbrella, staffing (including issues of credentialing of CAM practitioners) and reimbursement (insurance coverage of CAM has only recently begun to improve).

Realizing the need for education to break down barriers created by unfamiliarity with CAM, the program has developed initiatives for medical students, residents and fellows. A one-month fourth-year elective in CAM has been highly popular through its eight year history; however, one of the greatest hurdles to getting into the core medical school curriculum has been finding time in an already overfull curriculum. The program now has lectures in all four years and is developing CAM curricula to be included in problem-based learning. One of the greatest benefits of the education program has been its contribution to humanizing medical education, bringing the emphasis back to aspects such as the therapeutic encounter and teaching self-care skills. Finally, through its Career Development and Training Program, the program is training the next generation of investigators who will ensure the future of high quality research in this field.

Complementary Therapies at the University of Pennsylvania

Alfred P. Fishman, M.D.
Senior Associate Dean, University of Pennsylvania;
Director of the Office of Complementary Therapies

On June 5, 1998, Dr. William N. Kelley, CEO/Dean of the University of Pennsylvania Medical Center and Health System charged a Working Group to deal with the question: "How does so-called 'Alternative Medicine' relate to our academic health center?" The procedure to be followed by the Working Group was to be identical with that traditionally used to assess the need for a new department or institute, i.e. successive reviews by standing committees of the faculty and administration.

The Working Group, made up of practitioners of "alternative medicine," clinical scientists and administrators met monthly over the next 9 months. At the half-way mark, the state of deliberations was presented at a retreat which included a critical audience of about

100 members of faculty, administration (both university and medical school) practitioners of medicine in the Penn Health System and nationally prominent leaders in health care policy. The recommendation of the meeting that the Working Group continue its assessment was followed during the next few months by presentations to the relevant departments and administrative offices. Three subgroups were created to deal with clinical practice, research and education. Questionnaires concerning the use of unconvential therapies were sent to 1500 physicians were in the Penn Health System and the 800 responses were included in the final report. The conclusions and recommendations were accepted by the medical faculty and administration and approved for implementation by the CEO/Dean.

The Conclusions and Recommendations fall into four categories: General, Clinical Practice, Education and Research. Key recommendations are the following:

I. General

1. The Academic Medical Center must continue to practice scientific (evidence-based) medicine.

2. Each unconventional therapy should be evaluated separately.

3. The designation "Complementary" is preferable to "alternative" since individual therapies, rather than systems of therapies will be assessed and usage will be complementary rather than alternative.

4. Traditional approaches for evaluating traditional western medicine will be applied to unconventional and unproven therapies considered for inclusion in the practice of conventional medicine.

5. A Steering Committee will be created to advise about program development, evaluate proposals and serve as advisory to the existing offices of Medical Affairs, Human Resources and Legal Affairs as well as to Heads of Departments, Centers and Institutes and similar entities.

6. An appropriate administrative structure will be created. (This has evolved into an "Office of Complementary Therapies" headed by Dr. Fishman, former Chair of the Working Group

and since Chair of the Steering Committee).

II. Clinical Practice

1. In evaluating the use of complementary therapies, distinctions should be drawn between harmless therapies and potentially hazardous therapies. Existing mechanisms for individual privileges should be applied. The process for evluating a proposed therapy should be basically the same for complementary therapies as for conventional therapies except for the addition of the Steering Committee as a reivew group.

2. The offices of Medical Affairs, Human Resources and Legal Affairs should perform the same functions for assessing competency in the various complementary therapies as for conventional medicine. Complementary therapies practiced in the UPHS should undergo review in accord with policies and guidelines developed by these offices. The Steering Committeee will serve in an advisory capacity to these offices.

3. Complementary medicine should be organized as a "virtual center" so that standardized practices could be accomplished at the different inter-linked sites.

III. Education

1. Medical students, house staff and practicing physicians need to be well informed about complementary therapies. Need exists to educate physicians about the nature and content of unconventional therapies that their patients are using and to instruct them to be critical in their use.

2. Instruction about complementary therapies should be part of the medical curriculum and available as electives. Instruction should be available for house staff and practicing physicians.

IV. Research

1. The same criteria and guidelines should be used for unconventional and conventional (scientific) therapies. Unproven therapies may constitute opportunities for research.

2. The Steering Committee should encourage research in complementary therapies. Advantage should be taken of opportunities

provided by the new Center for Complementary and Alternative Medicine of the National Institutes of Health, which is affording funds for such research.

3. The University of Pennsylvania Health System should encourage research into selected unconventional therapies. In doing so, advantage should be taken of the many opportunities for such training in clinical and basic science departments, in the Center for Clinical Epidemiology and Biostatistics, and the Department of Biostatistics and Epidemiology, in other components of the University, e.g. the Leonard Davis Institute, the Wharton School, and in various offices engaged in health services research.

Implementation of the above recommendations has been greatly expedited by the use of familiar, traditional and existing administrative mechanisms to create the program and to monitor its operations and efficacy in accord with standard health system guidelines. Equally important is the fact that faculty and administration were informed and involved throughout the deliberations that led to the adoption of the program and creation of the Office of Complementary Therapies.

Research in Complementary Therapies at the University of Pennsylvania

Brian Strom, M.D., M.P.H.*
Chair of the Department of Biostatistics and
Epidemiology and Director of the
Center of Clinical Epidemiology and Biostatistics
University of Pennsylvania Health System

Dr. Strom chaired the focus group concerned with assessing the role of research on complementary therapies. The group was initially skeptical about adopting unproven and unconventional therapies and took as its charge the appraisal, from a research perspective, of how complementary therapies might be incorporated into the

* The following is a synopsis of a longer presentation made by Dr. Strom at the meeting.

academic health system. Starting with the proposition that many practices in medicine were found not to work as expected when finally subjected to testing, the group agreed that the issues concerning CAM were the same as those that faced conventional medicine.

The consensus was that complementary medicine could serve in a complementary role in that it embodied alternative approaches for medical thinking and considered aspects of western life not dealt with by western medicine. As a working definition of complementary medicine, the group included therapies that had not been proven by clinical trials or did not derive from an understanding of the underlying physiology. Operationally, the group defined complementary therapies as those not normally used by practitioners of conventional western medicine.

Since all therapies involve potential and/or risks and potential and/or known benefits, the group recognized that good clinical management requires that the best information be used to balance risks and benefits and that information is often incomplete when decisions have to be made. The primary consumers of the research were identified not only as the scientific community but also included payers, politicians and the public. The topics for research have to be chosen in keeping with these consumers and effective means for reporting the results have to be established. Proper clinical research will enable sorting of unconventional therapies into those that should be adopted, thereby becoming conventional, and those that should be rejected. For such research to be conducted, standardization of therapeutic products and interventions is essential and the use of the therapies in a non-western belief system would have to be weighed in the balance. It is understood that each question would have to be addressed by individual design rather than by a blanket approach.

Key questions are those of safety and efficacy. Are there drug interactions with the herbal remedy? Other questions relate to costs, patients satisfaction, quality of life, predictors of response and immediate markers of the effects of therapy.

Studies of complementary therapies must be structured as carfully as those used for conventional clinical research, including comparable control groups. For complementary therapies as for conventional therapies, risk/benefit balances have to be carefully weighed.

Because of the prospect that some therapies currently regarded as complementary will prove to be safe and effective, the academic health center should facilitate research directed at evaluating unconventional therapies that seem promising.

The group called attention to the important distinction between the standard of evidence required by the individual provider recommending or delivering services to the individual patients and that required by a health system that is considering establishment of a program to deliver health care. The latter demands a higher standard of evidence concerning safety and efficacy.

With respect to introducing complementary therapies into the academic health system, the program should begin with a few therapies that have been proven or will be evaluated scientifically. For scientific evaluations, the studies should begin with a focus on short-term safety and efficacy. Careful acount has to be taken of short-term adverse effects which may affect future usage, including both toxicities and undue delays in conventional therapies. Before the study is about to begin, a careful review of pertinent literature should have been accomplished with particular reference to potential risks and hazard. The synthesis of the results of this review should be presented for institutional review by individuals not involved in providing the service.

Complementary therapy protocols for research should be reviewed in the standard way by institutional review boards. The research should be formal and not simply conducted by a clinician collecting data while delivering care. In essence, a clinical program devoted to complementary therapies should be identical with conventional scientific programs which recognize faculty effort devoted to the research, the programmatic needs in terms of time and resources for implementation, and careful institutional monitoring for safety and efficacy.

Also recommended is the recruitment of new faculty with a primary interest in conducting research in complementary therapies. For this purpose, a multi-departmental search committee would help to ensure acceptance by the faculty of the new personnel. Moreover, joint investment by the school, the relevant center(s) and the home department in the new faculty members and their research would greatly enhance acceptance of the program. In addition, a research training program in complementary therapies, funded by the school, would help to launch the research program. As a start, the evaluation process could begin with therapies that are widely used and likely to prove safe and effective. In turn, this initiative would be expected to result in extramural funding.

Because of financial restrictions, recruiting at Penn has been delayed. Instead, researchers and programs have been developed from within. A neurologist trained in Epidemiology has become interested in research on acupuncture and has received research support from the NIH. An internist has received an NIH grant to evaluate herbs for hypercholesterolemia. A pediatric gastroenterologist is conducting research leading to a Master's degree on complementary therapies in pediatric irritable bowel disease. An assistant professor is applying imaging techniques to the study of meditation. Application has been made to the NIH for research and education grants and for a center devoted to unconventional usages of hyperbaric oxygenation. Penn has learned that research in keeping with western scientific standards is feasible and practical and affords new opportunities for inquiring minds interested in optimizing health care.

Section III

The Present Scene

Usage Patterns — What's Happening Now

David M. Eisenberg, M.D.*
Beth Israel-Deaconess Medical Center

Terminology

The designation of CAM, an acronym for complementary/alternative medicine has been popularized by the National Center for Complementary/Alternative Therapies. It encompasses a diverse assortment of therapies. A list, used in two national surveys, included chiropractic, acupuncture, massage, biofeedback, mega-vitamins, homeopathy, relaxation and meditation, guided imagery, spiritual healing by others, self-help, commercial diet, folk remedies, hypnosis, lifestyle diet, herbal remedies, and energy healing; the latter, in the minds of respondents, meant laying on of hands and the use of magnets.

The Evolution of CAM in the United States

In 1992, the Office of Alternative Medicine was authorized. In 1993, *New England Journal of Medicine* published the first CAM survey and the NIH established the Office of Alternative Medicine. By 1995, the NIH had funded 10 centers of excellence. By 1998, the office was advanced to the level of a national center with an initial research budget of 50 million dollars per year. In 1998, Marcia Angell and Jerome Kassirir, in an editorial in the *New England Journal of Medicine*, pointed out that there was not enough science involved in CAM. A month later, the *JAMA* and all the *AMA* specialty journals were devoted exclusively to CAM; in all, 80 articles were published. George Lundbergh and in an accompanying editorial, Phil Fontanerossa declared that there was no alternative medicine; they recognized only good medicine and pointed out that it is the responsibility of the physician to distinguish between the good and the bad.

By 1999, the NIH had funded additional centers and its budget had increased. Pharmaceutical companies became involved, envisaging a 10 billion dollar industry, which would increase at 20-30 percent per annum in the United States. In 2000, the White House established the Presidential Commission on CAM Policy to examine the state of clinical practice, research and education in the United States and to recommend national policy for this evolving health profession.

---

* The following is a synopsis of a longer presentation made by Dr. Eisenberg at the meeting.

The Prevalence of CAM Usage

CAM usage in the United States is not confined to any single segment of the population; women use CAM slightly more than do men; African-Americans slightly less than other groups; people on the west coast slightly more than the other parts of the country. Usages differ by only a few percentage points, and are probably socially and demographically insignificant. Individuals under 30 years of age increasingly resort to CAM as part of their lifestyle.

European surveys have implicated "Baby-Boomers" among the highest users. However, in the United States survey, 30 percent of 311 respondents over 65 years of age used at least one complementary therapy for severe illness during the proceeding year. The two most popular therapies were chiropractic or herbs and vitamins. Both usages entail risks. Thus, the remarkable increase in CAM usage cannot be discounted as due to "Baby Boomers." Concomitantly, it can also be anticipated that those who are better educated and have a higher income will be part of this trend.

The movement is to more and more usage. In fact, during the past 12 months, there has been an increase in the percentage of Americans who use these therapies to treat serious illnesses. In 1990, there were more visits to alternative providers than to primary care doctors.

This growth was not because people made more visits per person but simply because more people made visits. At least 200 million more visits are being made to chiropractors, massage therapists, acupuncturists and the like than to all primary care physicians. A breakdown of 60 million visits indicates that half are for massage and chiropractic; chiropractic alone accounts for 200 million visits. Four therapies are used by at least 10 percent of adults in the United States: chiropractic, massage, herbal therapies and relaxation and meditation.

In 1997, out-of-pocket expenditures were exceptionally high in the following categories: all hospitalization co-payments, 9 million dollars; all medical doctor services 29 billion dollars; all CAM therapies and office visits 27-34 billion dollars. In essence the out-of pocket amount paid by the American public, for CAM is of the same order of magnitude as for all M.D. services.

About one in five of 200 patients that took prescription medications reported concurrent use of at least one herb or high-dose vitamin. This observation relates to recent disclosures of drug-herb interactions, probably in our most vulnerable populations, such as those with chronic or life-threatening illness, on multiple drugs, or with hepatic or renal insufficiency.

Notifying Their Physicians

The degree to which Americans reveal their use of these therapies to physicians did not budge from 1990, when 60 percent said they had not discussed it, to 1997, when the figure was 61 percent. There is an enormous communication problem. Conventional medicine has not created an atmosphere that would allow patients the freedom, the ability and the luxury, of feeling comfortable about telling a doctor or nurse about their use of unconventional therapies.

Authoritative data regarding the use of alternative therapy among minority populations is not available. The National Institutes of Health is preparing a proposal to assess this use by African-Americans, Hispanic Spanish-speaking people, and selected Asian populations because the patterns are clearly different. Generalizing from the previous surveys of white middle class Americans overlooks ethnic distinctions in the use of health care.

The same national data set included out-of-pocket expenditures by quartile of income: those in the highest income quartile spent about 500 dollars a years, while those in the lowest quartile spend about 265 dollars a year. Although it might anticipate that low income would be a barrier to CAM use nonetheless, 43 percent of those in the lowest income group – those making less than 20,000 dollars a year – spent at least 250 dollars out-of-pocket on CAM.

During the past 5 years significant endorsements of certain CAM therapies have materialized: AHCPR guidelines include chiropractic for acute low back pain: mind-body techniques for pain and insomnia; an NIH consensus conference has identified indications for acupuncture; evidence has been offered to support the use of moxibustion for breech presentation; psychosocial support for cancer patients has become almost commonplace. Whether psychosocial support alters quality of life or affects the natural course of illness is unknown.

The use of homeopathy is a controversial topic. Analysis in the medical literature from Great Britain – one in *The Lancet* and another in the *British Medical Journal* – create a conundrum; either homeopathy works or the randomized placebo control trial does not.

Major news articles and headlines around the world have featured a number of herbs including St. John's Wort for depression, ginkgo for Alzheimer's Disease, herbs for irritable bowel, saw palmetto for benign prostatic hypertrophy. The peer-reviewed literature contains at least as many negative studies as positive studies. Despite favorable publicity, randomized control trials need to be conducted.

Examples of the direct toxicity of certain herbs are becoming increasingly frequent. These include comfrey and chaparral, which can damage the liver. Ma huang (ephedra) and yohimbe possess catecholamine-stimulating factors which can be dangerous for those with cardiac arrhythmias. In *The Lancet* last December, St. John's Wort was reported to interact with theophylline, cyclosporine, warfarin, and estrogens, decreasing bioavailability and evoking clinically significant adverse events. St. John's Wort also interacted with SSRIs; yohimbe with tricyclics. In a separate study, St. John's Wort decreased the concentration of the antiviral agent used to treat AIDS.

Who is Practicing?

Richard A. Cooper, M.D. and Heather J. McKee, M.Div.
Health Policy Institute, Medical College of Wisconsin

Introduction

Throughout most of the 20th century, physicians were the principal providers of patient care, and patients experienced care principally within the context of the medical model. This role for physicians was favored by regulatory and reimbursement policies and by their sheer numbers, which, by the end of the century, reached more than 600,000[1]. However, as we enter a new century, physicians are joined by a growing cadre of other clinicians in a range of traditional and alternative disciplines.[2,3] While the scope of practice of these clinicians overlaps that of physicians, they approach the care of patients from a variety philosophic vantage points.

This review considers five such disciplines. Two traditional disciplines, nurse practitioners (NPs) and certified nurse-midwives (CNMs), grew out of nursing and bridge the medical and complementary models of patient care. Three others are the complementary and alternative disciplines of chiropractic, naturopathy and acupuncture. Practitioners in each of these five disciplines are licensed to take the principal responsibility for patients, under at least some circumstances, and each is growing substantially in both numbers and licensed prerogatives. Although both naturopaths and chiropractors are called "doctor" or "physician" in many states, we have applied the term nonphysician clinician (NPC) to these and the other disciplines discussed herein to distinguish them from allopathic and osteopathic physicians. Collectively, these disciplines represent an evolving force in health care.

This review begins with an assessment of the overall dynamics of health care spending and employment that have contributed to the growth of all of the health care disciplines. It continues with a description of the five NPC disciplines cited above and closes with a consideration of the future roles of physicians and NPCs in the context of evolving multidisciplinary systems of health care.

Economics and Health Care Employment

While many cultural, technological and political factors undoubtedly contribute to the utilization of health care services, the dominant factor is the economy. Therefore, before considering the disciplines that contribute to the provision of complementary and alternative health care services, it is useful to reflect on the economic milieu in which that health care is offered and purchased. Figure 1 depicts the relationship between the US economy, as measured by the per capita gross domestic produce (GDP), and national health expenditures, also assessed in per capita terms, over the period from 1960 to 1997. A striking correlation is apparent (R^2 = 0.95). Also apparent is the deviation of points above the line during the years from 1991 to 1996, a period during which health care spending was generally viewed as excessive. While, in inflation adjusted dollars, GDP per capita approximately doubled during this 37-year period, health care spending per capita increased five-fold.

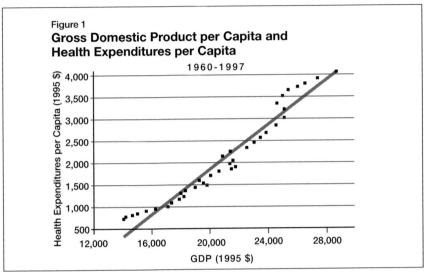

Figure 1
Gross domestic product (GDP) per capita and health care expenditures per capita
in the US, 1960-1997. Both are expressed in 1995 dollars. Data are from the
Organization for Economic Development and Cooperation (OEDC), 1999.

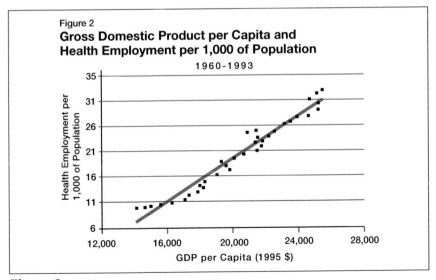

Figure 2
Gross domestic product (GDP) per capita (expressed in 1995 dollars) and health
employment per 1,000 of population in the US, 1960-1993. Data are from the
Organization for Economic Development and Cooperation (OEDC), 1999.

Health care is a labor-intensive-activity. Most health care expenditures are for physicians and other advanced clinicians, pharmacists, nurses and support personnel. Therefore as health care expenditures increased, it is not surprising that health care employment (expressed as workers for 1,000 of population) also increased (Figure 2). General employment also increased during this period of time, as more women entered the labor force, but the fraction of total employment that was devoted to health care increased even more, from 2.6 percent of total employment in 1960 to 7.0 percent in 1993.

These trends in the growth of health employment extend back to before the Civil War, and they are projected to continue. Figure 3b, which was adapted from the work of Kendix and Getzen[4], displays this phenomenon. While 150 years ago more than 90 percent of health care workers were physicians, they now account for less than 10 percent of the health care workforce. The greatest growth has been among the nursing, technical and support disciplines and more recently, among managerial personnel. Significant numbers of NPCs first became evident in the early 1900s, and over the past 40 years these disciplines have grown out of proportion to the growth in physician supply. The NPCs represented in Figure 3a include not only the five disciplines discussed herein but also psychologists, optometrists, podiatrists and nurse anesthetists.

Thus, for many decades, an expanding economy has enabled more health care spending, and this has been expressed principally as a growth in the health care workforce. What will the future hold? In a speech at the University of Michigan in 1999, Alan Greenspan, Chairman of the Federal Reserve, said "it is safe to say that we are witnessing this decade, in the United States, history's most compelling demonstration of the productive capacity of free peoples operating in free markets. The generations that follow are being bequeathed the tools for achieving a material existence that neither my generation nor any that preceded it could have even remotely imagined as we began our life's work." A significant manifestation of this material existence is health care. This reality is implicit in various governmental projections. For example, while the Bureau of Economic Analysis (BEA) has projected that per capita economic expansion will continue at two to three percent annually, the Health Care Financing Administration (HCFA) has projected that the growth of health care spending will exceed this by more than 50 percent, and the Bureau of Labor Statistics (BLS) has projected levels of health care employment that

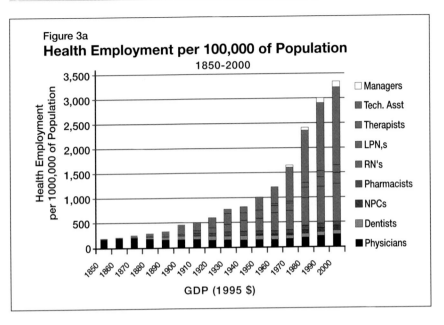

Figure 3a
Health Employment per 100,000 of Population
1850-2000

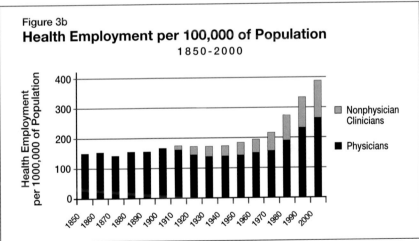

Figure 3b
Health Employment per 100,000 of Population
1850-2000

Figures 3a & 3b

Health employment in the US per 100,00 of population, 1850-2000. Adapted from Kendix and Getzen[4] and from the Bureau of Labor Statistics[5]. RN = registered nurse. LPN = licensed practical nurse. Tech Asst = technicians and assistants. NPCs = non-physician clinicians, including not only the five disciplines discussed in this report but also optometrists, podiatrists, psychologists and nurse anesthetists parallel this projected growth in health care spending[5].

It appears, therefore, that the public expects more health care and is willing to purchase it in proportion to the national wealth. Moreover, these expectations have grown from simply purchasing medical care to the medicalization of life's natural processes and the pursuit of perfect health[6]. One way that the public purchases health care is through personal spending "out of pocket," but most is through group or communal actions, such as employee benefits in lieu of wages or taxation, which distribute health care benefits more broadly. There is tension at the margin, as expectations exceed resources and as personal desires conflict with communal responsibility. Nonetheless, aggregate spending continues to grow in parallel with the economy. As is evident from the last 150 years of health employment, this growth creates a demand not only for physicians but for other health professions who supplement and complement the care that physicians provide and who do so not only within the context of the medical model of care but also through other healing philosophies.

Traditional Nonphysician Clinicians

Nurse Practitioners. NPs are the largest group of NPCs and the one that is undergoing the most rapid growth[3]. Their philosophic approaches to patient care, which are rooted in nursing, bridge the medical and complementary models of care[7]. NPs view patients from a holistic perspective, and they view illness within the context of the spectrum of life's stages. They focus on the wholeness of people and the interaction between people and their environments, emphasizing not only the treatment of disease but also the enhancement of comfort and general well-being, characteristics that historically have been associated with physicians, as well.[7,8] Thus, while scientific advances in medical care have been associated with a loss of the supportive and caring functions of healing that historically have been provided by physicians.[8] NPs have retained these elements as central components of their discipline.

The training of NPs, most of which is at the master's level, builds on their nursing education. It includes the care of acute and chronic illness across a broad spectrum of disease, with an emphasis on prevention, case management, counseling and patient education.[2] Most NPs train in various areas of primary care, such as adult health, pediatrics, family health, women's health or gerontology. However,

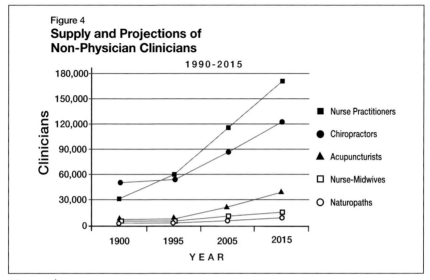

Figure 4
Supply and projections of nonphysician clinicians, 1990-2015. Data and projections are updated from previously published analysis[3].

small but increasing numbers of NPs are choosing careers in critical care, emergency care and other specialty pathways.

While in 1990 there were fewer than 30,000 active NPs, NP training programs have proliferated, and the number graduated annually has increased from 1,500 in 1990 to 7,500 in 1999. As a consequence, the number of NPs reached almost 90,000 in 1999, and it will surpass 115,000 by 2005, a number that is similar to the projected number of family physicians.[1, 3] Growth of this discipline is projected to continue.

Licensure for NPs is available in every state[2]. They are given significant latitude to diagnose and care for patients throughout the range of disease and dysfunction that falls within their training and expertise, including ordering and interpreting diagnostic tests and performing minor procedures.[3, 9] NPs may practice independent of physician supervision in almost half of the states, but some degree of physician oversight or delegation is required in the others. However, in many states, such oversight may be at intervals extending from a few days to several weeks, and some states permit even greater independence when caring for underserved populations. In addition, two-thirds of the states have granted NPs prescriptive authority for controlled substances, which, in many states, is independent of physician involvement. While licensed to practice independently, most NPs choose to practice with physicians. In that context, they take the major responsibility for patient education, wellness care, the care of minor and self-limited disorders, and counseling in areas such as life style, nutrition and emotional health. Randomized studies indicate that disease outcomes are equivalent whether patients receive care from NPs or physicians.[10] However, satisfaction is generally greater when care is provided by NPs. Patients placed a particularly high value on the time that NPs allot for counseling and communication.

Certified Nurse-Midwives. CNMs come from a background of nursing but enter the separate discipline of midwifery.[11] By definition, their training is focused on obstetrical and gynecological care, family planning, counseling and patient education. Philosophically, they are rooted in traditions of holistic medicine and the care of disadvantaged and underserved populations. They believe that women are well designed for pregnancy and childbirth, they avoid interfering with the natural process, and they encourage breast-feeding. Whereas the medical model often substitutes technology for the use of professional time, midwifery care is time intensive. For example, it calls for hands-on assistance throughout labor. However, the health and safety of the mother and baby are not the CNMs' only goals. They value childbirth as an emotionally, socially and spiritually-meaningful life experience that has the potential to strengthen the bonds within a family and promote the personal growth of all of its members.[11]

The licensure and prescriptive privileges of C.N.M.'s parallel those of N.P.'s.[2, 9, 12] Their prerogatives include the authority to care for normal pregnancies and perform normal deliveries in all states, provide non-pregnant gynecologic care in most states and care for complicated pregnancies in many. Most states require that CNMs maintain a relationship with an obstetrician and consult when deemed necessary. Although several states allow them to care for patients independent of any requirement for physician collaboration, the traditions of midwifery call for collegial relationships with physicians.

Nurse-midwifery is a small field, but it is growing. In 1990, there were 3,000 CNMs and they attended almost 4 percent of all births (Figure 4).

By 1997, that number had doubled to 6,000, and the proportion of births attended by CNMs grew to 7 percent.[13] At current training levels, there will be approximately 10,000 CNMs in 2005,[3] and they can be anticipated to attend more than 10 percent of births. While in 1995 the ratio of CNMs to obstetricians was 1:6, that ratio will fall to 1:4 by 2005.

Alternative Nonphysician Clinicians

Chiropractors. Chiropractic is the most established of the alternative disciplines. It is built around the "chiropractic encounter," which emphasizes physical contact with patients and the stimulation and support of natural processes.[14] The goal of chiropractic education, which spans four years, is to prepare chiropractors to be primary care providers who can serve as the portal of entry to the health care system, performing wellness care, general primary care and musculoskeletal care. They are expected to diagnose and care for patients in health and disease and to consult with or refer to other health care providers when necessary.[14] Their training concentrates on disorders attributable to the neuromusculoskeletal systems, with an emphasis on chiropractic technique. Although only 10 percent of their clinical training is specifically devoted to other organ systems, chiropractors also care for a range of viscerosomatic disorders, often ascribing their etiology to a neuromusculoskeletal basis.

Chiropractors are licensed in all of 50 states, and they are regulated by separate boards of chiropractic in 48.[2,15] Few practice in large urban areas with populations of greater than one million, and most are in towns of less than 100,000, a distribution that is reciprocal to that of physicians.[16] In 1990, there were 50,000 chiropractors (Figure 4). This number grew only modestly during most of the 1990s, reaching 60,000 in 1998, but the number of graduates more than doubled to 4,400 in 1998 despite the fact that no new colleges were established.[17] Enrollment has receded over the past two years, but an additional college recently opened and another is planned. Given these countervailing trends, the future is uncertain. Conservative estimates suggest that the number of chiropractors is likely to reach 85,000 by 2005 and to exceed 100,000 by 2015.

State practice acts have given chiropractors broad and independent latitude to diagnose and treat "disease" or "physiologic dysfunction" by means of manipulation, physiotherapy and other physical means in all states. They also may give dietary advice in all states and use therapeutic massage in most. Indeed, approximately 80 percent of chiropractors report that they utilize nutritional counseling and massage in their practices. They also have the authority to prescribe and dispense minerals, herbal remedies and food supplements in most states, but this prescriptive authority is limited to natural products and does not include controlled drugs. Several states allow them to serve as "gatekeepers," and managed care plans in some of these states have delegated that responsibility to them.

The neuromusculoskeletal (NMS) role of chiropractors is directed principally to disorders of the spine and limbs using manipulation and other physical modalities. Collectively, these disorders account for 85-90 percent of patient volume.[16] While chiropractors use a range of physical modalities in treating NMS disorders, spinal manipulative therapy (SMT) is the major modality and the one that most characterizes the profession. Outcomes studies in patients with low back pain indicate that symptom control is attained with SMT. However, the overall efficacy of chiropractic SMT is similar to that of spinal manipulation provided either by osteopathic physicians or allopathic physicians, physical therapy, massage therapy, medical treatment provided by either family physicians or orthopedic surgeons or brochures explaining self-treatment, alone or in various combinations.[18-20]

A second but smaller arena of chiropractic treatment is for viscerosomatic conditions, such as otitis, asthma and hypertension. These account for 10-15 percent of chiropractic visits. Some viscerosomatic disorders are chronic, but others are acute and self-limited. Both adults and children are treated. However, not all chiropractors provide this care, and there is division within the profession between the "straights" and the "mixers" concerning the appropriateness of its inclusion in chiropractic practice. Nonetheless, through changes in state laws and regulations, the chiropractic profession has sought to broaden its authority to treat these disorders. Yet, such treatment is not well supported by outcomes research, and its effectiveness has been questioned. Moreover, even physicians who refer patients with NMS syndromes to chiropractors tend not to refer patients with viscerosomatic disorders, and private insurers commonly exclude reimbursement for these conditions.

In recent years, many chiropractors have expanded their treatment repertoire to include acupuncture, and some have adopted other alternative treatment approaches, such as massage and herbal therapy. Thirty states permit chiropractors to perform acupuncture, and nineteen permit them to practice homeopathy. Efforts continue to extend state practice acts to permit the broader use of such modalities. At the same time, other practitioners, including physicians, are employing manipulation in their own practices. In addition, although most osteopathic physicians appear to have gravitated into the allopathic realm and largely abandoned manipulation, the surge of interest in spinal manipulation has prompted the osteopathic profession to re-examine the role of manual therapies.[21] Interest in manipulative therapy is also growing among allopathic physicians, particularly in the specialties of physical medicine and family medicine, and among physical therapists. However, for these other disciplines, manipulation is usually adjunctive to other therapeutic approaches, whereas chiropractic SMT is generally the primary intervention. In response to this widening interest, the chiropractic profession has sought to limit reimbursement for SMT to chiropractors, both through changes if regulations within HCFA and through legislative action in a number of states.

One of chiropractic's strongest characteristics is the high degree of satisfaction expressed by patients. This appears to relate not simply to the perceived outcomes of manipulation and other therapeutic modalities but more broadly to the "chiropractic encounter," which includes both personal interaction and physical contact with each patient.[22] These characteristics have also been associated with the practice of medicine, although the prevalence of their use appears to have waned.[8] The void created invites the participation of other practitioners, and chiropractors appear willing to serve this role.

Acupuncturists. Most practitioners of acupuncture and herbal medicine provide care within the tradition of Chinese medicine, which emphasizes an empirical, holistic approach to prevention and the restoration of balance.[23] Like other alternative NPCs, acupuncturists are trained to be the clinicians of first encounter. Their curriculum, which usually spans three years, prepares them to approach diagnosis from the Oriental perspective (look, smell, listen and feel) and to treat pain, addiction and other common disorders with acupuncture and/or herbal remedies. In most states they earn a master's degree from accredited schools, but some schools award certificates. At present there are 43 accredited schools of acupuncture and nine others awaiting accreditation. Their total enrollment exceeds 5,000. While most are based on traditional Chinese medicine, in which acupuncture and herbology are linked, other forms of acupuncture are taught and practiced, including Japanese acupuncture, Korean hand acupuncture, French auricular acupuncture and French energetic acupuncture.

Acupuncturists are licensed in only 35 states.[2,24] Approximately half hold a master's degree and half have certificates or diplomas. Seventy percent practice alone or in acupuncture groups, but 30 percent practice in multidisciplinary settings, usually with other alternative practitioners. Most states allow them to practice independently, but some require the involvement of a physician, dentist or chiropractor, and 10 states require referral from a physician. Acupuncturists are authorized to diagnose disease and dysfunction and to treat using needles and energetics. In more than half of the states, they are specifically permitted to prescribe and dispense minerals, herbal remedies and food supplements. Indeed, almost all practitioners report that they recommend herbal remedies, and 85 percent dispense them. In addition, some states permit acupuncturists to practice homeopathy.

In 1990, there were approximately 5,000 licensed acupuncturists. By 1997, that number had grown to 11,000. However, with the recent expansion in the number of acupuncture schools, the number of acupuncturists is projected to grow, exceeding 25,000 by 2005 and to reach more than 50,000 by 2015 (Figure 4).[3] These projected numbers could be even greater if licensure spreads to the remaining states, as seems likely, and additional training programs are established to serve these regions.

Two-thirds of patients who seek care from acupuncturists have musculoskeletal complaints, and a large number have headaches, fatigue, depression and related symptoms. Approximately 70 percent are female. Acupuncture visits are characteristically long, usually exceeding one hour. While patients receiving acupuncture often see a physician or other clinician for the same disorder, acupuncture is the major or only modality in almost half of the cases. It is likely that the future use of acupuncture for these and other disorders will be influenced by the a 1997 NIH Consensus Conference, which endorsed the use of acupuncture in a range of circumstances, including painful musculoskeletal syndromes, fibromyalgia, osteoarthritis, postoperative pain, drug addiction, stroke rehabilitation, headache and asthma.[23]

Naturopaths. Naturopaths take a holistic approach to healing that emphasizes the stimulation and support of natural processes.[25] Like allopathic and osteopathic physicians, they receive four years of post-baccalaureate education culminating in a doctoral degree. Their education spans the pre-clinical sciences and the clinical disciplines, with an emphasis on health promotion, prevention and treatment based on the stimulation or support of natural processes. Included are training in herbal medicine, nutritional medicine, acupuncture, homeopathy, hydrotherapy, mind-body medicine, massage and natural childbirth.[25] Some obtain added certification in acupuncture, traditional Chinese medicine or midwifery. Their clinical education, which is entirely outpatient-based, is designed to prepare them to be primary care providers. However, their licensed scope-of-practice and traditions exclude many of the drugs and procedures that are commonly used by primary care physicians, and their spectrum of practice is, therefore, much narrower. In addition, not all practicing naturopaths received training of the breadth and scope indicated above and not all practice in states with licensure laws.

Naturopaths are licensed in only eleven states, but several others are considering licensure.[2,26] Only Utah requires an additional year of residency training, although graduates in other states often seek such training.[25] All states that license naturopaths consider them to be physicians and designate their titles as "Doctor of Naturopathic Medicine" (ND) or "Naturopathic Physician" (NP). They are allowed to treat common diseases using manipulation and other physical modalities, herbal remedies and other natural substances and non-controlled drugs. Most states also permit them to provide obstetrical and gynecological care, suture wounds and perform minor invasive procedures, and some permit them to serve as "gatekeepers." In general, these practices are independent of physician supervision or delegation.

The usual scope of practice of naturopaths includes disorders such as arthritis, chronic fatigue, headache, irritable bowel, upper respiratory infection, vaginitis and symptom control associated with chemotherapy, but it generally excludes diseases of greater severity, such as congestive heart failure, acute abdomen, GI bleeding, stroke and chest pain. Thus, naturopaths tend to concentrate their care toward the least complex end of the spectrum of primary care.

The number of naturopaths is quite small. In 1997, there were only

1,400 in the eleven states that license naturopathy (Figure 4) and approximately 500 others in the states that do not currently offer licensure.[3,17] However, two new naturopathy schools opened over the past several years, bringing the total to four, and additional schools are likely. Therefore, the total number of naturopaths is projected to reach 4,000 by 2005 and almost 8,000 by 2015[3] (Figure 4).

Reimbursement

Access to reimbursement enables NPCs to function as autonomous health care providers. Therefore, it is not surprising that state and federal laws assuring reimbursement have been vigorously sought by the NPC disciplines. In 1977, the Rural Health Clinics Act provided the first direct Medicare and Medicaid reimbursement for NPs and CNMs, but it was limited to those working in freestanding, physician-directed rural clinics located in health professions shortage areas (HPSAs). This was subsequently expanded to cover other locations, and on-site physician supervision was waived unless it was a requirement of the state. The Balanced Budget Act of 1997 further expanded direct Medicare reimbursement for NPs to include all non-hospital sites, and it removed any requirement for physician involvement in states that had no such requirement. Chiropractors are the only alternative NPCs who are reimbursed by Medicare, but that reimbursement is limited to SMT for the treatment of subluxations. They also are reimbursed under workman's compensation, and half of the states reimburse chiropractors under Medicaid. In contrast, none of the governmental payers currently cover acupuncturists or naturopaths.

Many states have enacted laws mandating that private health plans include reimbursement for one or more of the NPC disciplines. In addition, a number of states have enacted "any willing provider" (AWP) laws that, in general, prohibit health plans from denying access to any licensed provider whose training and scope-of-practice includes the services covered by the plan and who is willing to meet the terms and conditions of the plan. Most such laws are broad in their definition of providers, although some cite specific disciplines. State courts have overturned or limited the AWP laws in several states, based on conflicts with the Employee Retirement Insurance Security Act (ERISA). However, a provision of the federal Patient Protection Act, recently considered by the Congress, would mandate that all health plans include NPCs among their providers if the benefits covered in the plan are within their scope-of-practice of those disciplines. This would greatly strengthen the access of NPCs reimbursement. However, even in states that lack these various mandates, reimbursement for NPCs, particularly those in the alternative disciplines, is increasing in response to consumer demand from enrollees and employers.

Multidisciplinary Care

As is evident from the foregoing discussion, there is considerable overlap between the scope of practice of physicians and NPCs and substantial overlap among NPCs. In recent years, a number of organizational factors have evolved which create opportunities for these various professionals to engage in collaborative practices that extend the range and quality of care available to patients. For example the economics of health care have encouraged the development of group practices in which patient care responsibilities can be distributed among disciplines. The skill and compensation levels of various providers can be matched to the services that are needed, and multiple practitioners can bring together complementary treatment modalities. This is further encouraged by studies that have found that the care of both the traditional and alternative NPC disciplines is generally cost-effective and is met with a high degree of patient satisfaction.[10,11,18,21,27] As a result, provider organizations, such as clinics, hospitals and health maintenance organizations, are incorporating increasing numbers of NPCs into their systems of practice.[28] At the same time, insurers are creating benefit plans that include both traditional and alternative NPCs, partially in response to state mandates but also in response to consumer demand.

The second organizational reality that has created opportunities for NPCs to engage in collaborative practices is time, or, more accurately, the lack of time. Historically, western medicine was rooted in traditions that wedded empiricism and humanism. These traditions, which first came together during the 4th century BC under the teachings of Hippocrates, found expression during the early 20th century in teachers such as Francis Weld Peabody, who observed that an interest in humanity, which is one of the essential qualities of the physician, requires the lavish expenditure of "time, sympathy and understanding."[29] Unfortunately, medicine's remarkable transition from empiricism to science during the 20th Century has had the unintended consequence of dampening the expression of medical humanism. Many have observed that the current systems of medical education have largely failed to adequately equip physicians with the tools that they need to feel equally comfortable with the quantitative distinctions of scientific medicine and the ambiguities of human emotion.[8,30] Moreover, recent changes in health care financing have further eroded the ability of physicians to devote the time necessary to practice humanistic medicine, as power has shifted to insurance companies, managed care organizations and federal bureaucracies and as productivity has become paramount in physician practices. While the NPC disciplines discussed herein have not escaped from these same realities, lavishly dispensing time remains the hallmark of each. Indeed, each has a healing culture that is rooted in natural medicine and that views the time spent with patients as essential to the healing process. These characteristics have created enhanced opportunities for collaboration with physicians. Indeed, the blending of skills and philosophies that can result from such collaborations has the potential not only to enhance patient care but to strengthen the health care system over all.

References

1. Cooper R.A.. Perspectives on the physician workforce to the year 2020. *JAMA.* 1995;274:1534-1543.

2. Cooper R.A., Henderson T., Dietrich C.L.. Roles of nonphysician clinicians as autonomous providers of patient care. *JAMA.* 1998;280:795-802.

3. Cooper RA, Laud P, Dietrich CL. Current and projected workforce of nonphysician clinicians. *JAMA.* 1998;280:788-794.

4. Kendix M., Getzen T.E.. US services employment: A time series analysis. *Health Economics.* 1994;3:169-181.

5. Braddock D. Occupational employment projections to 2008. Monthly Labor Review., 1999; November:51-76.

6. Goodwin J.S.. Geriatrics and the limits of modern medicine. *NEJM* 1999;340:1283-1285.

7. Baer E.D.. Philosophic and historical bases of advanced practice nursing roles. In Nurses, Nurse Practitioners: Evolution to Advanced Practice. M.D. Mezey and D.O. McGivern, eds. New York, N.Y.: Springer Publishing Co., Inc. 1999, pp. 72-91.

8. Pellegrino E.D.. The sociocultural impact of twentieth century therapeutics. In The Therapeutic Revolution: Essays in the Social History of American Medicine. M.J. Vogel and C.E. Ewards, eds. Philadelphia, Pa. University of Pennsylvania Press. 1979, pp. 262-263.

9. Henderson T, Fox-Grage W, Lewis S. Scope of Practice & Reimbursement for Advanced Practice Registered Nurses; A State-by-State Analysis.. Washington, D.C.: Intergovernmental Health Policy Project, George Washington University. 1995.

10. Mundinger M.O.. Primary care outcomes in patients treated by nurse practitioners or physicians. *JAMA.* 2000; 283:59-68.

11. Rooks J. Midwifery and Childbirth in America. Philadelphia, PA: Temple University Press. 1997.

12. American College of Nurse-Midwives. <u>Nurse Midwifery Today; A Handbook of State Legislation</u>. Washington DC: American College of Nurse-Midwives. 1997.

13. Curtin S.C., Park M.M.. Trends in the attendant, place, and timing of births, and in the use of obstetric interventions: United States, 1989-97. Nat. Vital Statistics Reports. 1999, Number 27.

14. American Chiropractic Association. Chiropractic State of the Art. Arlington, VA: American Chiropractic Association. 1994.

15. Federation of Chiropractic Licensing Boards. Official Directory, Chiropractic Licensure and Practice Statistics. Greeley, C.O.: Federation of Chiropractic Licensing Boards. 1998.

16. American Chiropractic Association. Annual Physician Survey and Statistical Study. Arlington, VA: American Chiropractic Association. 1994.

17. Cooper R.A., Stoflet SJ. Trends in the education and practice of alternative medicine clinicians. *Health Aff* (Millwood). 1996;15(3):226-238.

18. Carey T.S., Garrett J., Jackman A., McLaughlin C., Fryer J., Smucker D.R.. The outcomes and costs of care for acute low back pain among patients seen by primary care physicians, chiropractors and orthopedic surgeons. *NEJM.* 1995;333:913-917.

19. Cherkin D., Deyo R.A., Battie M., Street J., Barlow W. A comparison of physical therapy, chiropractic manipulation, and provision of and educational booklet for the treatment of patients with low back pain. *NEJM.* 1998;339:1021-1029.

20. Andersson G.B.J., Lucente T., Davis A.M., Kappler R.E., Lipton J.A., Leurgans S. A comparison of osteopathic spinal manipulation with standard care for patients with low back pain. *NEJM.* 1999;341:1426-1431.

21. Howell J.D. The paradox of osteopathy. *NEJM.* 1999;341:1465-1468.

22. Coulter I., Adams A., Coggan P., Wilkes M., Gonyea M. A comparative study of chiropractic and medical education. *Alternative Therapies in Health & Medicine.* 1998;4(5):64-75

23. National Institutes of Health. NIH Consensus Development Conference on Acupuncture. Bethesda, MD: National Institutes of Health. 1997.

24. Mitchell B. State Acupuncture Laws. Washington, DC: National Acupuncture Foundation. 1996.

25. Jensen C.B.. Common paths in medical education. The training of allopaths, osteopaths, and naturopaths. *Alternative and Complementary Therapies.* 1997;5:276-280.

26. Alliance on State Licensing, Division of the American Association of Naturopathic Physicians. State Naturopathic Licensing Summary. Seattle, WA. The American Association of Naturopathic Physicians. 1997.

27. Hamric A. Outcomes associated with advanced practice nursing prescriptive authority. *J. Amer. Acac. Nurse Pract.* 1998;10:113-118.

28. Dial T.H., Palsbo S.E., Bergsten C., Gabel J.R., Weiner J. Clinical staffing in staff- and group-model HMOs. *Health Aff* (Millwood). 1995;14(2):169-180.

29. Peabody F.W.. The care of the patient. *JAMA.* 1927;88:877-882.

30. Magraw RM. Science and humanism: Medicine and existential anguish. In <u>Hippocrates Revisited</u>. R. Bulger, ed. New York, N.Y. MEDCOM Press. 1973. pp.43-49.

Cultural Diversity

Charles K. Francis, M.D.
Charles R. Drew University of Medicine and Science

I work at a medical center that is in the center of Watts, a hospital that was created to serve a diverse minority population. And having been at Drew in the early 1970s, returning to the East Coast for over 20 years, and then coming back to Drew, I find there's been a dramatic change in the diversity of the population we serve and, I think, a much more prominent use of complementary and alternative medicine in those patients.

I want to give you, first, a sense of just what diversity is in Los Angeles. As you know, Drew has a joint program with UCLA, so we attend both the Drew graduation and the UCLA graduation. The chaplain at UCLA did a marvelous thing last year and this year. At the end of the graduation ceremony, he asked students in the class to come up and give a greeting in the language that they speak at home. For each year, about 20 different languages have been represented in the graduating class at UCLA. Many of those students are Drew students.

At Drew, we have a population of students that is about one-third African American, one-third Latino, and one-third Asian and other, so that the population at Drew is very diverse. Having come from Harlem Hospital in New York City, where complementary and alternative medicine is also very prominent, it is clear we don't necessarily understand differences within populations. All Hispanics are not the same. Also, all African Americans are not the same.

We have mentioned the role of economics, and especially health insurance, in health care seeking behavior and I think that applies to complementary and alternative medicine as well. So I want to show you how insurance data impact on the distribution of health conditions that underserved populations have and how that might apply to the whole question of complementary and alternative medicine.

The background is fairly straightforward. The racial and ethnic disparities in American health care are increasing as the population is impacted by new immigration patterns, insurance status and lack of access to care. Health care providers, educators and public policy- makers have the opportunity to improve patient care through enhanced health professional education, patient education and, most importantly, the delivery of culturally competent health care.

A quick look at the demographics in Los Angeles from the 1997 census reveals that Los Angeles differs widely from the US in its diversity, with only 34 percent white compared with 73 percent in the US. Latinos in California, with 44 percent, are, by far, the largest segment of the population, compared with about 11 percent nationally. The African American population is relatively small, 12 to 13 percent nationally, but only nine percent in Los Angeles. Asian-Pacific Islanders, now with 13 percent, make up the fastest growing population in LA. Los Angeles also has the highest concentration of Native Americans living in urban settings of any city in the country. In that context, there is a challenge, first, to understand the diversity, and then to understand how it affects our health care delivery system and the kinds of programs we offer.

Also, it is a very young population, with 15-44 years the dominant age group (48 percent). There is not a very large number of elderly. at present, but of course that number is going to grow. Those data pertain to Los Angeles County, which differs from San Diego County or Orange County, where there are larger numbers of older individuals. We have a large proportion of people in the younger, childbearing age groups, with large numbers of Latinos and many young people in the school system.

What are the characteristics of this diverse population? One-third of them were born outside of the United States. And in contrast to 20 years ago, when most of Latinos were of Mexican origin, many now are now coming not from Mexico but from Central and South America. So there are differences from the Mexican population, many of whom are third or fourth generation Angelinos by now, compared with new arrivals from Central and South America where there are entirely different health care practices.

The Asians used to be largely from China, the Philippines, Korea, and Japan. There is a Korea Town, but there has been a dramatic change in the Asian population and now there is also Little Vietnam in one of the suburbs of Los Angeles. So we have a shift in the relative distribution of Asians, where new arrivals are coming from places other than China and Japan as they had traditionally done. And, of course, the Southeast Asian population from Vietnam and Cambodia has increased steadily. There has been a dramatic change in those Asian populations since 1980.

When we talk about what we want to do with alternative medicine, we are really asking a very difficult question in Los Angeles. Do we know the differences between Korean medicine and Vietnamese medicine? Spanish and African American medicine? It is very challenging if we are going to try and educate our students about what's going on with many of the patients we do see now; and we will be seeing increasingly diverse populations as time progresses.

National data show that in the 65-74 age group and the 75-84 age group, African Americans have the highest death rates, higher than for Asia-Pacific Islanders and even for American Indians and Hispanics. When people die early from diseases, their deletion skews the data later on in the lifespan. The data for men shows that essentially the same thing applies to African Americans in the other age groups, having the highest death rates at relatively early ages.

Indeed, age-adjusted mortality rates show African Americans have dramatically higher, overall adjusted mortality rates than the white, Latino, and Asian populations. Interestingly, the Asian death rate is the lowest of all of those groups. There has been significant improvement in the rates for the white population and some improvement in the total. Latinos actually have increasing death rates. But the rates for African Americans are still dramatically high, even though they are improving slightly as well.

In trying to understand this, I went back to David Eisenberg's work and found the baseline data fascinating. He noted that there is very little information on ethnic and racial minorities.[1] Herbal medicine, massage, self-help groups, mega-vitamins, healing energy, homeopathy, the major folk remedies, alternative and complementary therapies were found in that sample, and most commonly were used for chronic back problems, anxiety, depression and headaches.

Interestingly, use is more common among women than men, but less common in African Americans. Use is more common in the middle-age groups, so that older and younger people use alternative medicine less commonly. Use is also more common among those with a college education than without. Use was more common among those with higher income, and more common in the West.

Alternative and complementary medicine is basically a self-care process. People make the independent decision to take control of their health care and administer to themselves, using remedies that are available over the counter and do not require a physician. But they pay out-of-pocket, so that's where the economic factors come in, especially since most are not covered by health insurance.

How does that impact the populations in Los Angeles? Clearly there has been an increase in use of CAM.[2] In one survey the use of herbal remedies increased 380 percent and vitamins by 120 percent. My wife's gynecologist prescribed five megavitamins for her: thus he is a physician practicing alternative and complementary medicine; we are seeing more and more of that.

But the fact is that there are very few data on the use of complementary and alternative medicine among minorities. To quote David Eisenberg, again "parallel surveys modified to include therapies unique to minority populations and translated, when appropriate, should be conducted." Clearly there is a need to get a better handle on what the actual practices are in very diverse populations.

Some data come from a study on alternative and complementary therapies used by women with breast cancer in four ethnic populations.[3] These were data from San Francisco, studying the use, types and prevalence of conventional alternative therapies among Latino, African American, white and Chinese women diagnosed with breast cancer. Interviews were conducted by telephone. Fifty percent of the women in the study used at least one type of complementary or alternative medicine, one-third used two types, usually for less than six months. There are relatively well-established and effective therapies for breast cancer, but nevertheless a large number of these women used alternative or complementary medicine.

There were clearly racial and ethnic differences in use patterns. African Americans most often used spiritual healing, Chinese more often used herbal remedies, Latinos most often used dietary and spiritual healing while whites used dietary supplements or physical methods like massage and acupuncture most commonly. So across this relatively small spectrum of racial and ethnic diversity there was a wide array of choices of complementary and alternative medicines.

When we think about what we are going to teach our students, it perhaps should depend on the population that is being served by our respective educational institutions. What we may want to teach students about spiritual healing in Harlem may differ from what one would want to teach students in Phoenix, about spiritual healing among African Americans, and definitely from what one would teach about spiritual healing in Mexican Americans, [who employ a different type of spiritual healing].

Compared with the earlier data from Dr. Eisenberg, this group was younger, had higher educational levels or income, private insurance, exercise, and attended support groups.[4] Fifty percent discussed complementary and alternative medicine with their doctors, which is a surprising number because very often patients don't reveal that they are using alternative therapies. And, indeed, most of them felt that the therapies were helpful.

Another interesting study concerned home remedies. That was a national survey of African Americans with over 2,100 patients that looked at a different set of determinants of use of alternative therapy.[5] There was a tendency for alternative and complementary therapies to be used more often if the father had over 12 years of education; with lower educational levels, families tended to use these therapies less commonly. Religion was very important and correlated with the use. Living with a grandparent while growing up also was important.

Obviously the people who designed this study knew something about African American traditions. When I was growing up, I had a grandparent, but we also had someone we thought was a witch, who lived with us in my grandmother's house and who was a complementary and alternative medicine practitioner. We all came to Cousin Belle when we were sick and she would minister to us, give us teas and potions, and she lived in a little room all by herself, with kettles brewing and all kinds of things. Much of what my grandmother's nine children and all of us — 30-some — grandchildren know about health care, we learned from Cousin Belle.

Rural residence clearly correlated with increased use. In contrast to some general studies where these therapies were used more commonly in the western US, this was a study of African Americans in the south-central states. As we'd like to say it, people from "down-home" tend to use these therapies much more commonly.

Individuals in this study provide an interesting comparison to the earlier data. Females used CAM more commonly than males, and had lived with a grandparent when growing up. Lower educational level correlated with increased use in this population. Also, lower socioeconomic status, at least in this group, correlated with increased use.

But it was interesting that if one moved to the city — that is became a non-rural resident — the use of these therapies persisted as as if one had remained in the rural residence. And if you were poor in the city, you tended to use them more. I think it is the case that the poor people in New York and Los Angeles tend to use these therapies more commonly than people who grew up, perhaps, in non-rural or rural areas.

What about insurance? Many members of the population that we are serving, both majority and minority are uninsured. Work published in *JAMA*[6] shows the Hispanic population makes up the largest proportion of the uninsured. In educating young physicians or other health providers about alternative therapies, it is important to know what population one is dealing with, what proportion is insured or uninsured, as well as what the ethnic and racial diversity is.

In the uninsured population, there is a wide range of conditions that seem to be impacted by whether or not the family has insurance. So it is important to know, in a large uninsured population, how these diseases might be impacted by the use or lack of use of complementary and alternative medicine. Smoking is obviously much more common, obesity very much more common, as are hypertension, diabetes mellitus, elevated cholesterol and HIV risk. (There is some evidence that one can affect cholesterol levels with transcendental meditation).

A report recently put out by Los Angeles County (see tables 1-4 on following pages) shows the percentage of adults without insurance is highest in Latinos, then Asians and African Americans, and then white. The report also shows:

— African Americans smoke more often, but smoke less cigarettes, perhaps because of cost.

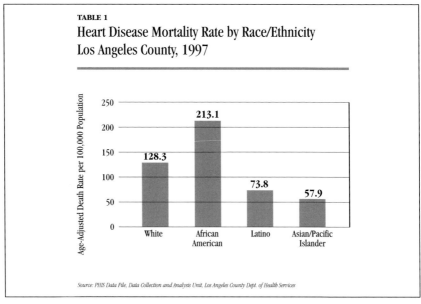

TABLE 1

Heart Disease Mortality Rate by Race/Ethnicity Los Angeles County, 1997

Source: PHIS Data File, Data Collection and Analysis Unit, Los Angeles County Dept. of Health Services

— Heart disease mortality is strikingly higher in African Americans, compared with Latinos and Asian/Pacific Islanders.

— Diabetes mortality, again, is highest in African Americans and much less common in Latinos and Asian/Pacific Islanders.

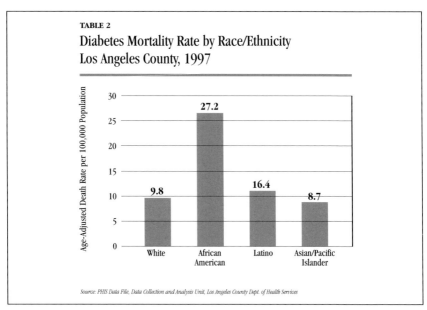

TABLE 2

Diabetes Mortality Rate by Race/Ethnicity Los Angeles County, 1997

Source: PHIS Data File, Data Collection and Analysis Unit, Los Angeles County Dept. of Health Services

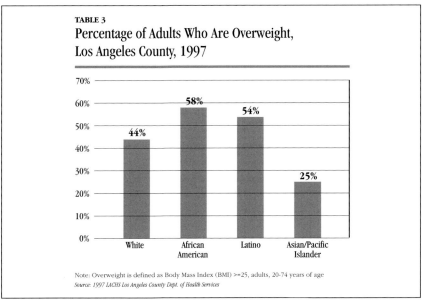

TABLE 3
Percentage of Adults Who Are Overweight, Los Angeles County, 1997

Note: Overweight is defined as Body Mass Index (BMI) >=25, adults, 20-74 years of age
Source: 1997 LACHS Los Angeles County Dept. of Health Services

— African American and Latinos are certainly more overweight compared with Asian/Pacific Islanders.

— Advanced cerebrovascular mortality is very high in African Americans, compared with Latinos and Asian/Pacific Islanders.

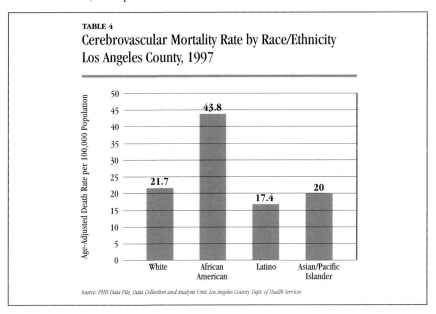

TABLE 4
Cerebrovascular Mortality Rate by Race/Ethnicity Los Angeles County, 1997

Source: PHIS Data File, Data Collection and Analysis Unit, Los Angeles County Dept. of Health Services

— It was uncommon to find adults who did not excersise in the
white population, in contrast to African Americans; and lack of
exercise in Latino populations was dramatically more prevalent
in males as well as females.

For African Americans, especially, I wanted to get a sense of the role
of religion and spirituality. I found one interesting paper that made
the point that the melting-pot idea, in the context in which we are
speaking, may not be entirely accurate. Most of us tend to hold on
to those traditional alternative and complementary medicine practices that our grandmothers told us about, and perhaps use them in
conjunction with mainline medicine, but the melting-pot does not
work in terms of how our home remedies or other health care
approaches are perceived.

It is important to keep in mind that there is heterogeneity within cultural
and ethnic groups. Having recently moved from New York to California,
I might even say there are differences in the African Americans on the
two coasts. In Harlem, we were all from Virginia and the Carolinas,
from the coastal southeastern states; and in Los Angeles largely from
Oklahoma, Texas, Arkansas: suggesting that there are, perhaps, different regional health beliefs within ethnic groups.

We need to understand the knowledge and impact of religion and
spiritual beliefs. Do we know how those things work, particularly
among Hispanic and African Americans? We should because it can
help health care professionals design interventions that are culture-
specific to the beliefs of individuals.

Educationally, programs are needed to increase the appreciation of
the extent to which diverse medical practices and beliefs shape the
lives of patients and influence health care behaviors. This is important when you think, particularly, about dealing with the diverse
ethnic groups we have here. You really don't know what's going on
in those neighborhoods, unless you deal with them often and regularly. Even though Columbia is only 3 miles from Harlem, you really
need to live in Harlem to get a feel for what the people in there are
experiencing and how these practices shape their lives.

Systematic knowledge of complementary and alternative medicine is
needed by practitioners, and I think, most importantly, research is
needed to determine the extent and nature and impact of complementary and alternative medicine, used among diverse and racial
and ethnic groups.

I want to mention, briefly, our programs at Drew with transcendental meditation. The Maharishi University in Iowa is collaborating with Drew on a number of issues. One is on stress reduction and atherosclerosis and cardiovascular disease in Blacks. Another involves basic mechanisms of meditation and cardiovascular disease in older African Americans; and a third, concerns the effect of herbal antioxidants on cardiovascular disease in older African Americans.

A recent report discussed the effects of transcendental meditation on carotid atherosclerosis in hypertensive African Americans[7]. The results show that carotid intimal medial thickness measurements predicted post-test carotid disease, but that stress reduction with TM reduced carotid atherosclerosis compared with no medication.

References

1. Eisenberg, D, *JAMA* 1998; 280; 1569-1575
2. id at 1
3. Marion L, et al. J.Nat'l Cancer Inst. 2000; 92:42-47
4. Ayanian, JZ, et al. *JAMA* 2000; 284; 2061-2069
5. Boyd, EL, et al. *J Nat'l Med Assoc.* 2000; 92:341-353
6. id at 4
7. Castillo-Richmond A, et al. *Stroke.* 31 (3): 568-73, 2000.

Cultural Competency

Dyanne D. Affonso, Ph.D., R.N.
University of Nebraska Medical School College of Nursing

The increased diversity of American society has evoked a national mandate for a culturally competent health professional workforce. National shifts in cultural diversity coincide with increased CAM use by the American public. Differences among the American population are also captured within the differences of CAM techniques used and preferred by racial and ethnic groups. Thus the concept of cultural competency affords another perspective for understanding the phenomenon of increased CAM use in the US.

To set a common frame of reference: two concepts, culture and competency, are examined when merged to form a health mandate of cultural competency. Although different views of cultural competency abound, definitions articulated by the HRSA Office of Women and Minority Health were selected for this presentation:

— Culture: patterns of human behaviors that include language, thoughts, communications, actions, customs, beliefs, values and institutions of racial, ethnic, religious or social groups.

— Competence: capacity to function effectively within the context of cultural beliefs, behaviors and needs presented by consumers and their communities.

— Thus cultural competency is a set of congruent behaviors, attitudes and policies that come together in a system or agency that enables effective work in cross cultural situations.

I propose that cultural competency is rooted in three domains that must be addressed in health care services: congruence, context and customize-tailor.

Congruence relates to the consistency and match between the health provider and person, or persons, to be cared for. Typically this is referred to as cultural-ethnic match based on commonalities relative to heritage, identity, backgrounds and lifestyles. Competencies associated with cultural-ethnic match are linguistic in nature, specifically language proficiency (as mandated by the Health Care Fairness Act of 1999), and a knowledge of cultural groups (awareness of beliefs, values and philosophies of a group different from the self). Cultural-ethnic match pertaining to CAM is commonly viewed as health providers who understand the cultural orientation of a given technique — acupuncture and Chinese medicine, self-healing aspects of meditation and Yoga.

However, another aspect of congruency, that of acculturation, continues to perplex health professionals because its impact and consequences are less understood, as is evident by the unfavorable outcomes that perpetuate health disparities. For example, it is documented that expectant Latinas who migrated from Central and South America and Mexico tend to have higher incidence of unfavorable pregnancy outcomes than their counterparts in the original country. In addition, Latinas generally have low health services utilization rates of prenatal care in the US, but high participation in CAM therapies.

We have yet to explore whether CAM is more congruent to the lifestyles of migrating Latinas in the US than standard prenatal care services. Therefore, competencies related to acculturation are not yet known and must be developed as investigations reveal the nature of exposure to the dominant American culture, including possible effects of separation from the original cultural heritage.

Another element of congruence involves "cognitive match" that relates to thoughts, beliefs, perceptions and expectations. Competencies related to cognitive match include awareness of different worldly views, learning about diverse cultural frameworks, and adapting to another perspective. Cognitive match is important to understanding the increased use of CAM, not only among racial and ethnic minority groups but also to grasping the worldly views of Anglo Americans who have gravitated to CAM despite their easy access to standard medical services. The majority of CAM users are not disillusioned by standard medical services, but rather they seek alternatives that are more congruent with their views and lifestyles.

Context is another quality of cultural competency, as cited by James Kelly: "Context is not just something; it is the heart and soul of the matter." Context implies coherence and provides meaning of events and experiences. Contextual competencies are reflected by the ethical principle of respect for persons that motivates health professionals in adapting to differences and similarities in the provision of health services.

Cultural competency is reflected by appreciation and acceptance that there are different ways of knowing. This means that knowledge takes on different characteristics, as articulated by Ernest Boyer in his book *Scholarship Revisited*. Boyer identified four domains of scholarship: Discovery (seeking new knowledge); integration (searching for new intellectual patterns to further knowledge); application (applying knowledge to serve the public); and teaching (communicating knowledge to future scholars).

These different domains of knowledge lead to a better understanding of CAM's increased use by the American public. Health professionals who accept that the process of knowing occurs within a context that is different from medical facts about a CAM technique are demonstrating cultural competency. However, busy health professionals largely overlook context in the delivery of health care services. We have yet to understand the impact of what people believe they must do to stay healthy and how values regarding self-care promote self-efficacy. In addition, we need to determine to what degree these contextual influences operate in the selection of CAM as a preference over standard medical services.

The third component of cultural competency is to individualize care by customizing and tailoring health services for different groups. "Customize" refers to planning and building according to specifications and "tailoring" implies adapting to specific needs. In the context of cultural competency, customizing is viewed as designing services based on people's needs and preferences; tailoring refers to complementing existing services with distinct styles of caring. Competencies by health professionals that reflect these two dimensions are demonstrated by the offering of ethnic specific services (targeted to different groups) and delivery of culturally specific interventions (appropriate across cultural groups).

Cultural competency as highlighted by congruence, context and customized-tailored services is important in building a culture of diversity within the health care system. A culture of diversity is rooted in varied approaches for comprehensive and integrated services. This culture offers a variety of interventions that gives deference to people's options, choices and preferences. Such a culture serves all persons from varied lifestyles, racial-ethnic heritages and urban-rural settings.

A culture of diversity accepts different ways of knowing, in understanding that the people's ways are typically communicated via CAM techniques. However, this culture of diversity is dedicated to scientific approaches in addressing issues of patient safety, ensuring protection from harm and bringing forward new data to better understand the people's motives in use of CAM. Thus, building the culture of diversity serves as a pathway to bridging the people's ways with the best of modern medical/health services.

A major objective of operating from a culture of diversity within a culturally competent health care system is the provision of cultural care. Cultural care is defined as services congruent with the beliefs, values and customs of the people to be served and operates within the context of the people's lives.

Four themes of cultural care highlight the interface between CAM and culturally competent health care. First is the integration of cultural scripts that make salient the beliefs of people in invoking pleas for help and other resources during health and illness. An example of a cultural script is the Hispanic "Milagros" which are small miracles in response to the use of charms and imagery as pleas for help during suffering and offering of gratitude for healing and recovery from illness. The competency relative to CAM involves identification of cultural scripts endorsed by CAM users to understand how CAM techniques provide helping resources in coping with health and illness experiences.

Another theme of cultural care is the use of metaphors to uncover the meanings experienced by people during health and illness. A salient example of the use of metaphors in health care is the cultural meaning of symptoms and causal attributions for diseases. Metaphors are powerful communication tools that have yet to be fully understood by health professionals. The relevance of metaphors to CAM is salient when exploring possibilities of what CAM might mean for the American public. First, CAM could be a metaphor for loss of hope (diminished belief) in standard medical services. Second, CAM, particularly meditation and contemplation, can be seen as a metaphor for self-healing. Third, CAM might be a metaphor for the diminished patient-provider relationship occurring in the managed care system.

Access to cultural healing systems is another theme of cultural care. This theme demonstrates cultural competency in appreciation that recovery and healing are equally important to diagnoses and treatments. People need time to heal, and healing practices and rituals provide time for human contacts that offer caring through presence, touch, listening, counsel and support. Healing rituals communicate passion, compassion and dignity for the person. CAM techniques encompass these features of caring; many persons describe their CAM experiences in the context of their satisfaction and pleasure with the healing aspects of CAM practices.

The fourth theme of cultural care involves spirituality, defined as the interconnectedness of human emotions. Spirituality is a common theme in culturally competent health care services among diverse groups. Spirituality is the essence of meaning in human experiences and propels the person to transcend human conditions and vulnerabilities. Just as there is a "Spirit of Medicine" and a "Spirit of Nursing" in standard health care services, there is also a "Spirit of the Person" that is salient during CAM techniques. The person's spirit is made visible through such human emotions as courage, joy, fear, pleasure, suffering, humor, anger and hope. These human emotions are frequently an integral part of CAM experiences and are released or reconciled in the human spirit that is communicated by repeated access to CAM encounters.

In summary, an understanding of cultural competency provides insights into the phenomenon of the increase in CAM use among the American public. Exploration of health care services that are congruent between person and provider, and attention to contextual qualities and services that are customized-tailored to the people we wish to serve, can serve as a model for bridging the humanistic qualities of CAM with the scientific aspects of modern medical services. The goal is to promote quality of life through quality care, and to decrease health disparities by expanding the scope of traditional health care services with more options for complementary care via safe and effective CAM practices.

The Intersection of Culture and Complementary Medicine

Bonnie B. O'Connor, Ph.D.
Hasbro Children's Hospital, Providence, RI

Although complementary medicine and cultural issues in health care have largely been considered as separate topics, this separation is purely heuristic. In fact the two topics are overlapping and mutually inter-influential, both in the dynamics of daily life and social institutions and in clinical and educational relevance. Their curricular and conceptual separation — from each other and from the rest of the medical curriculum, through encapsulation in specialized modules or mini-courses — has helped to foster and perpetuate several erroneous perceptions and assumptions and has sharply limited the scope of our understanding, inquiry and capacity to apply relevant knowledge to improved provider-patient relationships and patient-responsive care.

Everything that is socially developed and learned is a part of culture. It is the entire non-biological inheritance of human beings. That means that the methods and technologies and philosophical stances of biomedicine and science are cultural products just as much as are those of ethnomedical and other CAM systems. It is culture that shapes, propels and ratifies production of knowledge in any society. Culture

182

carries both the knowledge that we have and the values by which we apply that knowledge in various situations. Culture supplies us, also, with our expectations about when we apply our knowledge, what we think the outcomes will be and how we judge what's going on.

Furthermore, definitions of health, illness and appropriate care are always culturally derived and are interwoven with broader values and goals in both the general cultural fabric and in individual lives. That means that, whatever the healing system, it encodes and promotes certain values and norms and omits many other possibilities. A cultural reading of biomedicine, equally as of complementary medicines and multiculturalism in patient populations, is essential to a comprehensive understanding of the complex and dynamic cultural and medical pluralism which are *de facto* features of the current social landscape in the United States and many other countries.

Responses to health challenges entail: cultural values regarding appropriate response to problems or difficult circumstances (e.g., ignoring, accepting, working through, "fighting"); how persons are defined in relation to self; how persons are defined in relation to self and others (e.g., dependent, interdependent, independent); what constitutes proper and reliable decision-making (e.g., individual, collective, elder-controlled, professionally mediated); what kinds of exposures (e.g., to natural elements, to specific foods, to spiritual influences, to information that may provoke strong emotions) are beneficial or harmful; and conceptions of the nature of persons and their physical, emotional, mental and spiritual aspects, among many others.

Religious and philosophical convictions also enter in, such as the Buddhist expectation that a certain amount of discomfort and even suffering are normative and to be expected in life; the Islamic acceptance that illness and other events of serious consequence are ultimately in the hands of God; or the Taoist view that "when things are permitted to take their natural course, they move toward perfection and harmony." All of those tend to shape health interventions and responses to illness. Many of these broader beliefs and values are not directly about health, but they do play a defining role in the ways in which people respond to health threats and compromises, and to the maintenance or restoration of desirable states of being.

Culture is, therefore, involved in every health encounter. That is something that needs to be part of the education of a health professional. In the conventional clinical setting, as well as in the office of the homeopath or curandera or in interfamilial or self-care, cultural factors are introduced to the healing encounter by all parties to the interaction — providers as well as patients and family members. Cultural differences in fundamental assumptions and in values and goals, as well as in knowledge claims and the means by which they are validated as legitimate, lie at the heart of the strain inherent in the meeting of biomedicine with both multiculturalism and complementary medicine.

Cultural norms formulate our definition and recognition of authority and this fact also is central to an adequate understanding of the issues at hand. The term cultural authority designates the consensually recognized right of persons or social entities to define what is actual, factual or real; what is important, moral and desirable in life; and by what principles priorities may reasonably be set and conflicts among them adjudicated. Because of its consensual nature, trust is a crucial component of cultural authority.

Also critical is this fact: matters of meaning and value are always matters of cultural authority. So, for example, the meanings of sickness, the nature and effects of particular treatments, and the value assigned to competing principles, competing priorities and relative risks always reside in this domain.

Disputed cultural authority is central in the current social struggles over both CAM and cultural pluralism: their impacts on medical research, education and practice, and on health care choice-making in patient populations. Examples of disputed cultural authority include, for example, biomedicine's rejection of the theoretical, mechanistic and evidentiary claims of many CAM systems. Alternatively one sees diminished public recognition of the warrant of medical and scientific authority to define and control all matters pertinent to health and health care. And finally, there is unwillingness in the CAM community to accede to biomedicine's frequent efforts to act as sole arbiters of the boundary conditions of what is relevant or required in CAM research and efforts at integration with biomedicine.

Disputed cultural authority is as important to recognize in this effort as — indeed is inseparable from — specific disputed knowledge claims (such as whether qi exists, the supernatural intervenes in the processes of disease and healing, or high dilution substances can affect biological systems). One could suggest that cultural differences might be, or ought to be, put aside.

I submit to you that if we really thought about what that meant, that is not what we'd want to do, mostly because it reveals the general way that we have approached this is to say, "If you'd stop acting so much like yourself and act more like us, we'd be a lot more comfortable with that. We could use ways of collecting, validating and interpreting information and meaning and behavior that we are all familiar with and that we are comfortable with, and know work. So we'd appreciate it if you'd cut it out and be like this instead." But that's not a model that is likely to work very well in either of these domains.

I am going to read a longer-than-usual quote that's very pertinent to these subjects. It is from the *Diaries of Benjamin Franklin,* 1784: "Savages we call them because their manners differ from ours which we think the perfection of civility. They think the same of theirs.

"...the Indian men, when young, are hunters and warriors; when old, counselors; for all their government is by the counsel or advice of the sages; there is no force, there are no prisons, no officers to compel obedience, or inflict punishment. Hence they generally study oratory; the best speaker having the most influence. The Indian women till the ground, dress the food, nurse and bring up the children, and preserve and hand down to posterity, the memory of public transactions. These employments of men and women are accounted natural and honorable. Having few artificial wants, they have an abundance of leisure for improvement in conversation.

"Our laborious manner of life, compared with theirs, they esteem slavish and base, and the learning on which we value ourselves, they regard as frivolous and useless. An instance of this occurred at the Treaty of Lancaster, in Pennsylvania, anno 1744, between the government of Virginia and the Six Nations. After the principle business was settled the commissioners from Virginia acquainted the Indians by a speech, that there was at Williamsburg, a college, with a fund, for educating Indian youth; and that if the chiefs of the Six Nations would send down half a dozen of their sons to that college, the government would take care that they should be well provided for, and instructed in the learning of the white people.

"It is one of the Indian rules of politeness not to answer a public proposition the same day that it is made: they think that it would be treating it as a light matter, and they show it respect by taking time to consider it, as of a matter important. They therefore deferred their answer till the day following: when their speaker began by expressing their deep sense of the kindness of the Virginia government in making them that offer.

"'For we know,' says he, 'that you highly esteem the kind of learning taught in those colleges, and that the maintenance of our young men, while with you, would be very expensive to you. We are convinced, therefore that you mean to do us good by your proposal and we thank you heartily. But you who are wise must know, that different nations have different conceptions of things; and you will therefore not take it amiss, if our ideas of this kind of education happen not to be the same with yours. We have had some experience of it; several of our young people were formerly brought up at the colleges of the northern provinces; they were instructed in all your sciences; but when they came back to us they were bad runners; ignorant of every means of living in the woods; unable to bear either cold or hunger, knew neither how to build a cabin, take a deer, or kill an enemy; spoke our language imperfectly; were therefore neither fit for hunters, warriors or counselors; they were totally good for nothing. We are not, however, the less obliged by your kind offer, though we decline accepting it; and to show our grateful sense of it, if the gentlemen of Virginia will send us a dozen of their sons, we will take great care of their education, instruct them in all we know, and make men of them'".

I use that quotation often. I think it illustrates something very important in the kind of enterprise that we are trying to engage in here, where we have very different constructions of what's going on, of how it ought to go on, and of who has what to offer to whom. An inability to take seriously the proposition of the Six Nations or to see it in it any potential for learning or discovery of genuine value to the dominant group is indicative of the kind of attitude that impedes cooperative efforts and genuine moves toward integration. Offers of integration that are unremittingly unidirectional have less to do with integration than assimilation or absorption. This applies to the meeting of entire cultures as well as to the meeting of those cultural subsets which are their healing systems.

I think it is no accident that the topics of multiculturalism and complementary medicine have simultaneously commended themselves to the attention of the medical establishment. They are, I believe, two sides of a single coin. Both phenomena arise from, and contribute to, pluralism in America and other societies.

If one's goal is to establish and maintain diplomatic relations among the multiple world views that these important social movements represent, then informed and productive response to each requires conscious awareness of an earnest effort to avoid what ran in the *Harvard Educational Review* in 1952, called "Cultural Encapsulation." By that was meant a particular stance of mind, inhabiting a defensive or protective cognitive stance, that defined all of reality according to one's own cultural assumptions, that minimized or denied the importance or value of cultural differences, that imposed self-reference criteria only in judging the behavior of the claims of others, that ignored or deprecated evidence that might tend to disconfirm one's own perspectives, that depended solely on one's own techniques and strategies to design and solve problems, and that disregarded or explained away one's own cultural biases.

It is apparent, when features are enumerated in this way, that cultural capsulation is another name for what we call ethnocentrism. In cross-healing system engagement, the same phenomenon has been called medicocentrism, largely because of the nature and the direction of encounters along a power-gradient; but the caveat applies equally to all of us, of all persuasions. There is nothing to be gained and much to be lost in both demonizing and romanticizing. Clinging to our blinders can only inhibit the scope of our individual and collective vision.

I also want to talk about language. One of my favorite instructive quotes from Raymond Williams is: "When we come to say we just don't speak the same language, we mean that we have different immediate values or different kinds of valuation or that we are aware, often intangibly, of different formations and distributions of energy and interest. In such a case, each group is speaking its native language, but its uses are significantly different, especially when strong feelings or important ideas are in question."

Most certainly in the dialogue about conventional and complementary medicine, as in cross-cultural negotiations in general, there are many important ideas and very strong feelings at stake. Maybe one solution to the communications issue would be an effort to establish a new language, a "creolized" conjoined language that can combine in novel ways to form new modes of expression and thought. Maybe we should see if we could do it.

The education and training of health professionals in and about CAM, if it's to be more than an exercise in the defense and maintenance of a professional status-quo, must encourage openness —

which is not identical with acceptance — to varied worldviews and to an alternative structure for medical thinking. It is neither necessary, nor necessarily desirable, for medical curriculum to include required courses in anthropology or the social sciences. But it is necessary to incorporate, in meaningful ways, a cultural reading of systems of belief, knowledge and practice. This would include biomedicine, a basic understanding of intercultural dynamics, a deep appreciation of experiences, viewpoints and self-identified needs of patients, and some discussion of the concept of pluralism.

As is evident, I am a pluralist, which means I endorse "a society in which a range of groups and claims are able to maintain autonomous standards or participation in a common or shared enterprise." I submit that not only adequate education in the principles of CAM, but also full realization of patient-centered or relationship-centered, patient-responsive care will depend on enhancing the capacity of medical education to develop clinicians and researchers with the attitudes, skills and knowledge base to draw productively on multiple models of health, illness and care as they formulate research questions, appropriate methodologies, clinical strategies and population-based prevention and health promotion programs.

That is an equal requirement of both cultural competence in health care and of truly integrated medicine. Each must incorporate multimodal understandings, varying cultural and philosophical perspectives, and lay as well as professional criteria for identification of needs, goals, problem definitions, desirable outcomes and the criteria for their identification and evaluation.

Issues of Access: Who is Paying (Summary)

Wade M. Aubry, M.D.*
The Lewin Group

A key issue confronting both insurers and consumers is the integration of CAM coverage into existing health benefit plans. Though a number of plans and HMOs do offer some CAM benefits - usually chiropractic - most patients pay for CAM services directly. As a result, pressure for more coverage is growing and health plans are

---

* The following is a synopsis of a longer presentation made by Dr. Aubry at the meeting.

searching for ways to respond.

As they seek ways to expand CAM coverage, health plans confront a number of practical problems. The major one may reflect their concern that offering coverage for CAM services could undermine coverage decisions applied to other services, particularly new and emerging technologies. Most plans pay only for services that are medically necessary; they generally exclude coverage for procedures and services for which there is not sufficient evidence to support use.

Yet plans are not consistent in the way they define medical necessity. Several surveys have shown not only considerable variation in the definition used by plans, but also that plans often don't adhere to their own definitions and published policies. In addition, in some plans the medical necessity determination is made by an individual, in others according to formal coverage policy set by a committee.

Most plans rely on randomized clinical trials as the gold standard for developing evidence needed to support coverage based on medical necessity. Even so, a number of procedures that have not undergone this rigorous scrutiny and are not supported by such evidence are routinely covered. Often this coverage has been "grandfathered" because plans have found it difficult to remove coverage once a procedure is established and accepted as a community norm.

A number of health plans — especially PPOs, HMOs and Medicare - are expanding coverage decisions and now include outcome studies and other evidence of benefit. Some have explicitly adopted the requirement that covered services must be shown to improve health outcomes. Often this judgment applies to situations involving experimental therapy, especially services which are costly or used in life-threatening situations when existing therapeutic options are limited. To reduce the potential for litigation, some plans have begun to support clinical trials, either establishing a plan-specific trial or joining an NIH sponsored clinical trial.

Recently Medicare has become more flexible in its coverage decisions. By definition, Medicare will not pay for services that are not reasonable and necessary for diagnosis and treatment, which, in practice, means Medicare covers only procedures established as safe and effective, not those which are experimental or investigational.

Yet, Medicare does cover some CAM practices. From its inception, Medicare has covered chiropractic spinal manipulation and has agreed to cover the Dean Ornish Lifestyle Program for Heart Disease. With most coverage decisions now made locally, Medicare has been flexible enough to include coverage of clinical trials and certain investigational devices through agreement with the Food and Drug Administration.

Despite pressure for expanded CAM coverage, many plans have been slow to respond even though a number of strategies could be employed. The most straightforward approach - integrating CAM coverage into the existing benefit structure based on empirical observation and a commitment to prevention - has not been widely adopted, presumably because plans fear such coverage could undermine other coverage decisions.

Two other approaches have received greater support. Some plans have started offering special benefits riders, either on their own or limited to clinical trials to promote research, a tactic that has the virtue of both conducting needed CAM research and gradually integrating CAM benefits that meet defined criteria into existing plans. A third possibility, now gaining wider acceptance, is to offer plan members access to a discounted network of CAM providers. This strategy expands access to CAM services without undermining coverage decisions, but at the same time does not provide direct coverage because the patient ultimately pays.

Efforts to extend coverage for CAM services highlight the need for more and better research on these procedures. Though more plans are finding ways to improve CAM coverage, if only through access to discounted networks, market pressures will force more direct coverage. While health plans find it easier to cover those procedures and services demonstrated to be effective, a process is needed to assess those that are promising but still lack solid research support. That process might involve clinical trials or an external review panel. Procedures with no supporting data would not be included in that process.

Section IV

Issues Raised by Interaction of CAM and Traditional Medicine

The Significance of Shame and Humiliation in the Doctor/Patient Relationship

Aaron Lazare, M.D.
University of Massachusetts Medical Center

We have heard some of the failures of traditional medicine, including biomedical approaches that traditional medicine often ignores the belief system, that traditional medicine often fails to be patient-centered, that we don't listen to patients enough, that we fail to appreciate the importance of a doctor/patient relationship.

I'd like to review one approach that addresses this situation. It really speaks to traditional medicine, but it can also help bridge the gap. In particular, I want to address overlooked aspects of a set of emotions experienced by both patients and physicians. The emotions, in particular, are shame and humiliation, but in my studies what's added to that are embarrassment and guilt. The four together are referred to as the emotions of self-assessment, as the emotions you feel when something is wrong with your sense of who you are. The intellectual roots of this are not psychodynamic or behavioral but come from sociology, social psychology and the individual psychology of the emotions.

Before I entered this field, I worked in a walk-in clinic at Massachusets General and was trying to understand where patients were coming from. I did studies of patient requests. What did they want us to do for them? Apparently, at least in psychiatry, there was no literature on this. There had been literature on expectations, which was different. We broadened the notion of a patient's perspective. What is their request? What is their expectation? What is their feeling? What are their priorities? What are their goals? What kind of relationships do they want?

And then we began to look at and change the traditional model of the doctor/patient relationship from one where the patient tells you what's wrong and the doctor then tells you what to do to one with a negotiator, which sounds like everyday-kind-of-stuff now, but wasn't then.

But what I want to talk about is the significance of shame and humiliation and the power of looking at this and the fact that it is considerably overlooked. I had this epiphany after spending a day on the beach talking with a sociologist. All of a sudden it occurred to me: this is very important in medical care. While on my vacation in Maine, I asked everybody who was walking, jogging or climbing mountains if they had ever felt shamed or humiliated by their physician. And everyone said, in effect, "Do I have a story for you!" And they remembered them with great vividness.

I came back to the medical school and gave the first lecture. I was chair of psychiatry then and the students didn't know what my interest was. I asked all the medical students in the first year to write down the most traumatic experience they had had as a patient. (They averaged 20 to 23 years old). Then I asked them to tell me, in rank order, whether this concern or the anxiety and the angst over it had to deal with a fear of the diagnosis, the prognosis, the inconvenience, the cost or the shame. The majority said it was the shame.

Then I came across a fortuitous study from *The Lancet* of 187 patients who asked to die. I would have predicted the pain was overwhelming and that's why they wanted to die, but instead it was a feared loss of dignity, which is equivalent to talking about shame.

Then, again, trying to find out if there was something of substance, I went to the patient representative office. That's where patients complain and where you try to help them not sue the hospital. The person who ran it was an English major, a very empathic young woman. We concocted the following experiment: for the next few months, every person who comes here is asked "Why are you here? What brings you here?" by a doctor or a nurse. And then when the patient is finished telling their story, they say, "and how did that make you feel?"

About a third of the responses had to do with the billing system, but all of the others concerned experiences of shame and humiliation. "I felt abandoned," "betrayed," "conned," "disappointed," "duped," "eliminated," and so on. Or, "we are less than human," "eliminated from the decision-making process," "experimented on," "like a bum or forgotten person," "a little kid." Others said things like "not treated with dignity," "told I was a cry-baby," "took my manhood away," "treated me like a child in a nursery." "as if I were less than human," "a leaf shivering in a tree," "a cow," "like a dog with a tail between its leg," "like a puppy in a kennel."

I invited a group of patients who had successfully sued for malpractice to come for an interview in my home one Saturday afternoon. A lawyer gave me the list and, with their permission. I asked them about their malpractice experience. For all but one, the final straw was the humiliation. "There I was lying on my bed, cut my... off. It was a mistake, and I was managing it as best I could, and then he came by on his high horse, and never once even said that he cared or that he was sorry."

So that really powerful information was coming from all directions. One of the overall thrusts of what I want to communicate is that when we talk about caring for the patient, I think it's too vague. It doesn't tell you what's going on. Even treating the patient with dignity doesn't tell you enough. I think to really understand caring and dignity, you can explain a lot by looking at the other side of those features, namely the experiences of shame and humiliation.

And even though you may say patients rarely have those experiences, there's something about those emotions. When you have them, you never forget it. It doesn't take that much. If you spend an hour with a patient and there's only one minute of humiliation, that's enough. So it's a pretty touchy and very important business.

Harvard puts on a primary care course every year and I have now been presenting a somewhat longer version of this lecture for fifteen years. The response is very different depending on the audience. I present it to medical students and they think it's sort of interesting. I present it to interns and they're too busy. I present it to doctors in practice, even five to fifteen years into practice, and they are totally engaged. It starts to make sense of a lot of their experiences.

I had the unfortunate experience five years ago of helping my daughter through her death. She had cancer of the breast at the age of 27 and died two years later. I remember sitting in her room and saying, "Jackie, tell me about the shame and humiliation." She was really a tough kid. She was angry, angry at her cancer. And she said, "Those son-of-a-bitch doctors and nurses. They come in. They don't knock on the door. They walk up to me and they start interviewing me."

Then she said, "Wait!" And sure enough, they came. She said, "Just watch this one, Dad." So I am sitting there and she really takes them to task. They say, "Hello Jackie." And she says, "I didn't get your first names." Then she went on. "Wait a minute. I still don't know what roles you have. Who is the doctor? Who is the nurse?" She talked to them as a way of getting even. And I was really proud of her.

Look what we do to patients, the names we give them. These are the names of diagnoses. Cardiac is an embarrassment and heart is a failure. Coronaries are insufficient. You are hypertense and your infarction is inferior. I saw a patient who said, "I had a big infarction. This was a superior infarction. And they are telling me it's an inferior infarction." Obstetricians are worse. "You have an incompetent cervix." Or "you are a habitual aborter." "You are barren." Psychiatry is not much better. "You are narcissistic, dependent, histrionic," *et cetera.*

Are we are dealing with psychopathology? Absolutely not! This is the psychology of everyday life and I have mentioned where the intellectual roots come from. A lot depends on which specialty you are looking at, which is rather interesting. There are some specialties that are more humiliating than others.

For instance in dermatology, everyone can see and shame has to do with being exposed. John Updike has an interesting passage. He had psoriasis and in something called *The Journal of the Leper*, he says, "I am silvery, scaly. Tons of flakes fall wherever I rest my flesh, my torture is skin deep. There is no pain, not even itching. We lepers live a long time and ironically, healthy in other respects. Lusty, though we are loathsome to love. Keen-sighted, though we hate to look upon ourselves. The name of the disease, spiritually speaking, is humiliation."

Or a comment by a Swiss lawyer who wrote a book about his dying. He didn't want surgery for cancer of the bladder. He said, "Perhaps my decision to refuse surgery is motivated by too much pride and arrogance. Cannot bring myself to submit to surgery that leaves me hollowed out like a dug-out canoe that floats along with no one in control, diminished and mutilated. In order to survive must now be allowed to become so absolutely overpowering, that one submits to all these indignities."

Pediatrics is, of course, the shame of the heredity that you have may passed on, or how you have neglected your child.

In psychiatry, how can I not have taken care of my mental health?

For a long time, there was a lot of shame over cancer. One would hardly ever see anyone "dying of cancer," people always "died after a long illness." That's getting better. And of course, cancer affects the wrong kinds of organ. Your breasts, your ovaries, your testicles, your prostate. And that makes it very difficult for patients.

Death is a shameful thing. Death means the doctor has failed. Someone from Great Britain said, "Americans think that death is optional." And so, in England, they are saying, "No, you have to die." We don't let this happen, do we?

We talked a little bit about the emotions. People think when we first present the emotions that the topic is something soft and mushy. Some emotions are really rather distinct and you can identify them in a point I am going to try to make. Having identified them, you have a choice as to what you want to do.

I call them the signal emotions. In psychiatry, we used to call anxiety a signal emotion, a signal that something about yourself is in jeopardy. It rises when people judge that their thoughts and behaviors are wrong, that they haven't measured up to some standards or goals; that their expectations are less than they think they ought to be. A person feels exposed, deficient, defective, incompetent, inadequate, a failure. It sends everybody notice. There are certain physical signs — blushing, lowering and averting gaze, avoiding the eyes, hiding one's face, collapsing, shrinking one's body, fear of abandonment, perseverate disruptive behavior. The reaction is to hide.

The worst kind of thing is suicide. Remember Admiral Borda? They discovered that he was wearing insignias and medals that he wasn't supposed to and, as *Newsweek* came to talk with him, he did the ultimate and put a bullet into his chest.

Basically you have a whole lot of options about what to do when you discover that you are ashamed. I remember my first major shame experience in college. It was October and I had never left New Jersey before. I came from an industrial, blue-collar town. I went to Oberlin College and had never been away from home. I went a hayride with this gorgeous, blonde girl from Kenosha, Wis., the first Christian girl I ever dated. And she turned to me and asked, "Are you an athlete?" I used to study all the time; I was a nerd. So I turned to her and I said, "Yes, I run track."

Now, I feel very strongly about not lying. I am a very honest person and I felt ashamed. So, what was I going to do? You have a lot of choices. You can hide. You can break off the relationship. But spring came and I was still dating her and the track team was out. So I took a more constructive course. I joined the track team. I won three letters.

I felt ashamed. Shame is like blood pressure. If it's too high, you can die from it: if it's too low, you can die from it. But to feel shame is to know there is a better side of ourselves. It's the *sine qua non* of humanity.

Humiliation is different, but they are cut out of the same cloth. Humiliation is personal and you feel that it is unfair. You feel power-less. You feel unfairly lowered, debased, degraded, brought down. It's very characteristic. I am very aware of the humiliation. I feel blindsided. It's sort of a delayed reaction. You do a slow burn. You don't sleep that night and then grudges form, vengeance. Your judg-ment is impaired.

Have you ever written a letter to that person who had humiliated you? You think it's brilliant. You really think it's good. And then — fortunately if your secretary doesn't mail it and you look at it three days later — you'll say, "Oh, my God! I am so happy I didn't send it." I write about the psychology of apology and I get a lot of business from people who send e-mails too quickly and come running to me and say, "How do I apologize for that?"

You never forget your humiliations. The synonyms are very important to understand. Humiliation assumes you are to be nailed to the cross, to be decimated, eviscerated, assassinated. Humiliation is tantamount to being murdered psychologically. The murder of the self; and that's why when people are humiliated, people commit murders. The antecedent to that was a humiliation.

Shame and humiliation is the topic of the greatest book: it's the topic of the Old Testament. God is humiliated all the time and then has to get even. Satan was the humiliated highest angel that fell off and now he is getting even for eternity.

Physicians are very shame-prone. We tend to be perfectionists. Life and death are at stake. Our education is often associated with humiliation. We feel inadequate that we haven't read the latest

New England Journal of Medicine. The public expects a lot of us. Malpractice suits and HMOs humiliate us.

I always gave this lecture before the coffee break. Then doctors would come up to me and tell me their stories. I began asking them to write their most humiliating experiences in their professional careers. Now I have about 350 such stories. And they are the most anguished, painful stories. They fall into categories: When I was a medical student, when I was a house officer, when I made a treatment failures, when I failed the boards, why I was sued for was malpractice, when I committed a faux pas, *et cetera.*

Some of the most interesting ones were when doctors became sick. The question was, "In your professional career, what was your most humiliating experience?" Your sickness isn't your professional career, but it is. Doctors perceive that as their professional career. And the stories are really quite anguished.

I'll read one or two stories to close.

This one poor fellow was ashamed over his illness but he couldn't see a doctor for fear that he would be a crock. "When I was a resident, I fell at a roller-skating party. While my wife drove me to a hospital emergency room, I asked if my ankle looked as bad to her as it felt. I was relieved when she said that it was badly swollen, ecchymotic and angulated. I really felt good! I didn't need to worry that one of my fellow residents would pronounce my ankle as fine and my trip to the emergency room unnecessary. It turned out, thank God, to be a trimalleolar fracture.

The same doctor said, "When I had been an attending for about five years, I noticed that one of my testicles was enlarged, firm and asymmetric. I examined myself in the shower for several mornings before I was able to call a urologist colleague. I feared not only testicular cancer, but also the shame of having a normal exam, and thus, having over-diagnosed myself. So I didn't, I wasn't ashamed. Now I have been cancer-free for five years."

The stories tear your heart out.

"When I was an intern at a city hospital, I hit a patient... He, like so many of the patients, was a chronic alcoholic and now had *delirium tremens.* His bed was in the hallway, the hospital beds being completely filled. The lighting was poor and I was having a terrible time getting an IV needle into a shaking arm while he swore at me and the world. Finally, he said: 'You are going to hit me, aren't you?' I agreed that was accurate.

"'Well, go ahead then.' And I did. I wound up and socked him on the arm, an arm larger around than my thigh. 'Feeling better now?' he asked. 'Yes,' I replied. But I didn't; I felt terrible, I feel terrible now even though it's 35 years since it happened."

Most of these stories are 20 years old.

I can still see Mr. W.'s face and Mr. W.'s arm. I can still see Mr. W., whom I came to like and respect, watching me with a sort of timely, pitying look. My shamely narration is mine alone; no one was with Mr. W. and me that evening.

The stories that came to me were all true confessions. There was a great sense of relief from the doctor. They would send it to me, leaving their business card. I would type them all up and send them the whole package so they would get a chance to see what other people had to say.

What does all this have to do with clinical care? I think if we can identify these emotions, in ourselves and in our patients, there are ways to be therapeutic. These are the things that keep people from being satisfied, that keep people from lying. To be shamed is to hide. To hide is to break appointments. To hide is to lie to the doctor. Lie about your medicines: enormous clinical implications for that.

And also, the doctors are the loneliest souls because there is no one to tell. Doctors ought to learn how to trust at least a small group of people, so they could share this and not wait until I give a lecture and a course where they mail these things in to me.

I am still struggling with how we tie shame and humiliation together with alternative medicine, but I imagine that patients are ashamed to tell the doctors why they are seeking alternative medicine. They might be ashamed to tell the other doctors what's going on. Patients often won't tell you what kind of medicine they are taking. I have yet to work through all the connections, but I do believe that, even in traditional medicine, this is an important unexplored area if we want to get to the issue of dignity in talking to patients.

What Matters
From the Patient Point of View

Alice Trillin*
Consultant

Some of you may be wondering why I am here. I have no medical credentials whatsoever. I am listed as the representative for the patient point of view, so I suppose some of you assume that I am someone who has had successful experiences with CAM and I am going to tell you about that. The other qualification I have is I have been an educator for most of my life, though not in medical education until very recently.

I think the reason that I'm here is that when I first met June Osborn, she mentioned that she was thinking about sponsoring this conference and she was asking me my feelings about alternative medicine, (which is what I used to call it). I told her that when I had lung cancer at the age of 38 and my husband was quite deep into trying to help me deal with it and someone mentioned alternative medicine, he said that his idea of alternative medicine was a doctor who had gone to Johns Hopkins.

I thought I should start with where I am. I'm very much a traditional patient. When I got suddenly very ill after being very healthy for 38 years, I went right to my upper East Side New York Hospital internist, got a chest x-ray and was operated on 10 days later. Soon after that, I got myself — on my own by the way, not encouraged by my doctor — across the street to Memorial Sloan-Kettering, where I have been treated, or at least followed, ever since.

Some of you who are young practitioners probably are at least a little put off by the story about Johns Hopkins, thinking that shows a bit of contempt. But imagine that you were a conventional doctor and a patient came in and said, "You know, I am really into therapeutic touch." I think that you should realize that your reaction to me, thinking that I am rather close-minded, is probably rather parallel to that of a lot of the conventional doctors who have been confronted with CAM.

We ought to start by understanding that from both sides there really needs to be a little more openness and understanding and I include myself in that. Let me tell you a little bit about why I was, and why

*Deceased 9/11/01

my husband particularly was so resistant to the suggestion of alternative medicine. I had a disease that was probably going to kill me. I had malignant lymph nodes in my mediastinum in addition to adenocarcinoma in my lung. I think almost everybody, including the doctors, probably presumed I would die. We got a lot of phone calls from people recommending apricot pits or some such thing. To us, and I think particularly to my husband, that was an indication that they thought I was going to die, so I might as well go to New Mexico or Arizona or wherever they were doing that.

A very close friend of mine called me about a year later and told me that her 12-year-old son had a neuroepithelioma the size of a grapefruit attached to his aorta, and that it was inoperable because it was so close to the aorta. He actually got right to Columbia-Presbyterian and went to a pediatric hematologist who was able to shrink the tumor and operate. The boy got chemo and he is now a 32-year-old poet. But during the course of this rather courageous and very difficult treatment, he got a lot of calls about apricot pits, too. I asked her, "What was the most difficult? What could I do to help her? What could we talk about?" She said those were the most difficult calls she got because they were presuming that her child was doomed. And it was so hard. She said, "What should I do?" I said, "Just hang up the phone. Go uptown."

Cancer is not like some of the other illnesses we were talking about. I also think it depends a lot on who the person is who has it. What I am really saying to any of you who are angry at me for making a little bit light of this is that you have to recognize who I am. I am a skeptic and I am a highly rational person, and for me to deal with my illness any other way than the way I did would be a betrayal of who I am. To me that's the worst thing that you can do in terms of treating your illness.

Now let me go on the other hand. There are things that I don't understand about what happened to me and there are things that I don't understand about what happened to other people. So I am going to just tell you a couple of stories.

A couple of years ago a book appeared called *Medical Miracles* and, much to my dismay, I found that I was in it. I was really angry because some guy had called me and interviewed me on the phone for a few minutes. He apparently had talked to my doctor and portrayed me in this book as somebody who had survived my illness because of my will to live and my enormous courage, which was, as far as I was concerned, garbage. I did not want to be put in that position. I was really, really angry.

However, I had to admit — even though publicly I would never say that — there was a part of me that wondered why I wasn't dead! I mean there was something kind of odd about what had happened. I had two little girls who were four and seven. I did say, in an article I wrote for the *New England Journal of Medicine*, that I thought that the idea that their father would have to take care of their shoes and dental appointments was really an incentive not to die. He's a great guy, but I wasn't sure he was up to that.

And a part of me thought that was true. And, of course, I always thought some strange, biological thing was going on because there were cancer cells wandering around my body if I had malignant lymph nodes. But the balance was obviously in my favor and whatever tipped that balance may be something I didn't understand.

The other thing was that I had an incredible doctor. I had a doctor who practiced therapeutic touch. He was the Director of Medicine at Memorial for years. I don't think he would call it that. He was the most traditional doctor you can imagine, but when he examined me he touched me a lot. He did an old-fashioned kind of real physical examination. I also got to him because I rejected or fired the first doctor I saw who was recommended to me by Lewis Thomas.

I went to Dr. Thomas' very own physician,* who immediately started to blame me for having had lung cancer. I never smoked. I later took a look at my hospital record and saw a few notes on the visit saying: "Patient gives the story that she never smoked." I actually put that in a little piece in *The Times* one day, years later, but he really could not accept the fact — talk about blame and humiliation — that I hadn't caused my own cancer. Like how could I even have this disease if I never smoked. It was a horrible experience. It was painful, it was humiliating and I was mad as hell. I got out of there and said I was never going back into that hospital again. Actually, I was directed to Dr. Myers and I gave it another shot. He was an incredible man.

---

* Years later, this same doctor was at a lecture I was giving for graduating radiologists. He came up and said, "That was really wonderful. Mrs. Trillin, I am so pleased to meet you." I said, " Well, you already met me, actually" and I told him the story of our first encounter. I said, "You almost caused me to never set foot in this hospital again." And it was great! It was a good moment. And he was humiliated.

Every summer, my husband and I go to camp. We go to a place called the Hole-in-the-Wall-Gang Camp in Ashford, Connecticut. It's for kids with cancer and blood diseases and some other odd — we call them orphan — diseases. I have been doing this for five years and the kids have the most orthodox medical intervention you can imagine. A lot of them had leukemia. A lot of them had bone-marrow transplants. The kids with hemophilia are "on factor" before we take them horseback riding. The kids with thalassemia are on pumps every night. I mean we are talking state-of-the-art medicine. We all know about the incredible advances with leukemia treatment.

On the other hand, I have read stories from their doctors and from their parents about what has happened to kids, sometimes, after 10 days of camp and how their physical condition has changed. I don't know what to make of those stories. They are all about magic, so I am giving you both sides.

But let me turn to the other part of who I am, which is not just a patient but an educator, and talk about how I think what I know as both a patient and an educator — and a lot of things I heard here — could really affect how we teach.

I was always a teacher interested in radical change, in teaching the hardest, most difficult students. I went to Wellesley, Yale and all those classy places and taught in a regular university. Then in 1967, I went to City College of New York, in Harlem, and asked to teach open-admission students. I was 28 years old and I didn't know any better. I took on the most difficult students that we had who were in a course on basic writing.

When I got there, they were only taught grammar because what we saw was that their writing was ungrammatical. So they were not allowed to read — that was before I got there. A very senior member devised the curriculum. They were not allowed to write until they had studied grammar for one semester out of a book. Now all kinds of research shows that doesn't work. But I fortunately went with a really brilliant woman, who was my best friend and mentor, who said, "We have to ask questions about what is basic before we decide what to teach." And that's what I want to get to today in terms of what we want to do.

What is basic? We decided that what was basic was not what

appeared to be their errors but what was underlying that. Why did they make those errors? A lot of research has been done and a lot of progress in the humanities, in the teaching of reading and writing, which all has to do with writing as a way of teaching people to think more clearly, to express themselves. Then the grammar comes as a sort of editing process. We totally changed the way we did it and we really got better about it, until they took away all our money and there wasn't any more remediation in City University.

I have also produced educational television for quite a few years. And have always, again, been interested not as a producer — I don't really care about producing television — but as a teacher. How can you use that to change? I did a series on the teaching of writing, on the arts, and I am developing one on history. But I also said to my academic consultants, who were always very distinguished, "what is the basic question when I teach kids about the arts? Do we want to teach them the history of art? Do we want to teach them criticism? What, what's the real question?" The answer, in that case, was: "We want you to look at art in a different way." When we talked about American History, I did the same thing.

But let's say we do that with the teaching of what this conference is about, complementary and alternative medicine. What do we come up with? What's basic? At the meeting of the Planning Committee we all agreed that CAM was not anything that could be taught in isolation.

What we are talking about is really changing the attitudes of doctors so they look at their patients inclusively in the context of everything that they are. That includes their beliefs, the kind of skepticism that I am going to bring, or the kind of embracing of the other extreme of alternative practices that some patients may bring, their cultural differences, their religious differences as well as the psychosocial issues and the psychological questions that have been raised. Where do they live? How much money do they have?

These are things that I know are being introduced into medical school and taught, but I think that even though it's not new, it is important to re-address this constantly. I think that under the pressures of all the technological advances, that the issue gets subsumed and pushed aside constantly because students wonder, "Why should I take this course when I really need to learn more molecular biology?" And that's a very good question. If I had a daughter in medical school I would be paying the tuition and I would certainly ask it, and I would expect my students to ask it of me.

So, what is basic? I was struck by Dr. Feinstein's paper. I think the issue that he was getting at is how can we change the way patients expect to recover. Maybe that's got something to do with what happened to me: the placebo — I hate the word placebo because it sounds like a phony thing but you all understand what it means. But what we are really talking about is the negotiation or relationship, the partnership, between doctors and patients. What we have talked about today is what changes in the patient. It is not just that the patient has higher expectations. It is that the patient becomes an active participant in his or her own care.

If I think anything is responsible for my being here today, beyond my children and magic or whatever, it is that I did not let anybody else control what happened to me. I had to be in charge. My husband never took that control away from me by telling me what he thought I should do. He was there to support me, but he did not take the lead. His role was always following and supporting. My doctors did the same thing. I have been very, very lucky in my doctors, except for that one guy. But he got his.

And so I think what we are talking about is not just respect and not just listening. All these things are given. They are very, very important. I hate the word "empower" because it's become a sort of cliché, but it actually does mean something. Patients have to be given the ability to participate and to get better, to be healed with the help of whatever technology, but also the most support from family, society and any alternative therapy they can get their hands on.

And I hope CAM is going to be tested and I hope we are going to find out that lots of them work. I know that Memorial (Sloan Kettering) is now using herbs to treat prostate cancer. There are doctors there who, five years ago, made fun of all this but who are now saying thanks to some of their patients. They must be more open, not to the sort of fuzzy "Let's be understanding", but to the efficacy and the potency of some of these treatments.

So, we want all of it to help us. We have serious illnesses and chronic illnesses. We can educate our young physicians, but not only about the content. I don't want them actually to learn to do therapeutic touch unless they really want to. I would not spend those hours in the curriculum on the actual specifics of teaching doctors to do those therapies because there are a lot of other people who probably do them very well. I would spend time on teaching them to embrace cultural diversity, all the therapies that their patients might have access to or be interested in, and having them learn how to make their patients active participants with them as partners in their own care. We can do a lot better. Even though we have been trying, as I know, for 35 years, there is still a lot of room for progress.

Safety Issues in Mixed Therapies

Lisa Corbin Winslow, M.D.
University of Colorado Health Sciences Center

Every presentation needs to start with a history slide — at least that is what they told me in medical school — so here's a brief history of medicine. Starts out 2000 B.C. I have an earache; here, eat this fruit. 1000 A.D. That root is heathen; here, say a prayer. 1850. That prayer is superstition; here drink this potion. 1948. That potion is snake oil; here, swallow this pill. 1985. That pill is ineffective; here, take this antibiotic. And now we are back. The antibiotic is artificial; here, eat this root.

But we know from David Eisenberg's data that not only are patients eating the roots, they are still taking the antibiotic. He tells us 97 percent of patients who reported that they were seeing an alternative provider for a certain condition also were seeing a medical doctor. So there is a huge gray zone of overlap which we call complementary medicine. Because patients are using both, safety is a huge concern about which we really have little data.

I can't make my point any better than Hippocrates (an "old dead guy"), who said it best: "First, do no harm." That is what pushes us in conventional medicine and that should also push us in our approach `to understanding and recommending and fielding questions about alternative medicine. Or, as a young live guy said: "Safety trumps efficacy."

I sent out a survey to physicians in the Denver area in 1998 and asked them all sorts of questions about their attitudes on alternative medicine. I asked the physicians if they were interested in learning more about alternative medicine, and over 60 percent said they did want to learn more. Why? It wasn't because insurance was covering it. It was mostly because they agreed with Hippocrates. They wanted to dissuade their patients from use if a treatment was unsafe or ineffective: seventy-seven percent of those responding said this was important. So the safety issues tend to be first and foremost in the minds of conventional physicians when they are interested in alternative medicine.

What are some of the myths we are dealing with? The first one that must be we overcome is "natural equals safe." When my patients bring this up, I tend to refer to bee venom and hemlock as examples they can relate to: they are very natural, but not very safe.

How many times have you heard on TV an ad for an herbal product where the announcer says "it's 100 percent natural, so it is 100 percent safe." Truth in advertising: it drives me nuts. I see a commercial for ginseng, and it only goes over all the positives and they always say, "It's 100 percent natural so it's 100 percent safe." They don't give any information about possible side effects, or about people who should not use it. On the other hand, FDA-approved medications are required to tell every little side effect, even those that are not statistically significant compared to placebo; what's a patient going to think?

And then there is the myth that because treatments have been around for thousands of years and untold generations of Chinese people have used those treatments and medicines, they have to be safe. This test of time does not take into account rare adverse effects. That's what one gets from postmarketing surveillance. It doesn't highlight delayed effects like mutagenicity, in particular. One of the people I collaborate with has done some work with hypericin and he says it binds to DNA in the nucleus. What does that mean for long-term?

And then test of time doesn't really tell about effects that require long-term usage as well. So, I think, these are a few myths that your patient will bring to you and other physicians will bring to you. You need to know the counter-argument. Safety of alternative treatments is, at best, a murky issue. In most cases, at present, we just don't know.

Prospective safety studies are rare, and prospective studies combining conventional with alternative treatments are particularly lacking, as are combinations of alternative methods. What one sees in the conventional medical literature are primarily case reports of alternative adverse outcomes, often reported by conventional physicians who are presumed to have a bias against alternatives. There are beginning to be some case reports which will hopefully lead to scientifically testing the hypotheses. For example: certain herbs are found to decrease the efficacy of chemotherapy.

Primarily the focus is on anecdotal case reports for toxicities and adverse events. Anecdote is poor proof, and especially for proof of harm. This does a disservice to the alternative providers because it evokes hysteria in the medical community. I give lectures to my alternative medicine elective students or residents every month. One of the lectures I give is on herbs and the other one is on advising patients. It's amazing to me how much they think, "Oh, chiropractic. Totally dangerous! You know, absolutely. Because didn't you hear? Rupture this and that." That's because all they have are anecdotes. I think it gets a little over-blown and the truth is hard to find. There are very few prospective studies of the safety of alternative treatments.

There's even less known about combining conventional with alternative therapies: there are so few data. I don't know if it increases or decreases adverse events, side effects, or efficacy. There is   indication that some of the herbs touted to help relieve the nausea and vomiting associated with chemotherapy actually decrease the efficacy of the chemotherapy or at least decrease blood levels, but it is not known if it affects outcomes or not.

So what are the sources of toxicity? Delay of conventional therapy can be quite toxic, although that is not a fault of the alternative therapy by any means. Often the loss of physician-patient relationship is highlighted. If you tell your patient, "Oh, that's just a placebo. A bunch of quackery," that is definitely going to hurt that relationship. The patient is still going to use the medicine, but now the patient is not going to tell you, and may come in later with some sort of an adverse event or toxicity. You'll think you did your job because you told them not to use it and think they are not using. That's a tremendous source of toxicity in and of itself.

The credentialing of providers is all over the map and that certainly can be a source of toxicity if you are in a state where you don't need to have a license or you don't need to be regulated in any way. You can go hang up a shingle and call yourself whatever you want.

After this meeting, you might want to go back and educate physicians that chiropractic is fairly safe. But if you send your patient to a chiropractor who is also dispensing herbs, you have added a therapy that might not be so safe to what you thought was safe, so you have to keep this in mind.

We also talk about psychological harm. The way I am thinking of it is what happens if a person is convinced religious or spiritual healing is the way to go and then has a remission. I had a neighbor who had remission of her ovarian cancer. She had big meetings where all her friends came and prayed for her. Very emotional but I thought, "Boy, if that comes back, she is going to feel so guilty. She is going to think: I didn't pray hard enough! It's all my fault." The net effect could be serious psychological harm.

And then of course, there's bank account depletion.

Direct toxicities bring me to the topic of herbal medications, because I think that is where most imformation exists. Congress passed the Dietary Supplement and Health Education Act in 1994. The FDA had heard a lot of reports about adverse events due to herbs and they reacted with a move to regulate. That threat set off a huge letter-writing campaign: health food stores got their customers to write their congressman. In fact more mail was received on that issue than on the Vietnam War.

And so what happened? The resultant Congressional legislation stipulated that for a product that purports to be a dietary supplement, and which includes an herb, it is not necessary to prove that it is safe. The FDA has to prove it <u>unsafe</u>. Nor is it necessary to prove it efficacious. There is no standard of quality control, and the only limit they put on is that if it is to be called a supplement, the <u>manufacturer</u> is not allowed to claim to cure <u>disease</u>, only to suggest an effect on a <u>symptom</u>.

In this, I think, nobody wins. Neither manufacturers nor the patients can say what the product is for. Instead of saying "take this product for BPH," it must be said that it improves men's urinary tract health.

Recently there has been a change in the definition of "disease." It was decided that if symptoms are associated with natural states such as adolescence and acne, or pregnancy and morning sickness, those conditions are more natural and expected. In that case they are not diseases.

Consumer Reports did a nice article on herbs back in 1995, but I think it is still an excellent reference for lay clinicians, and for patients as well. One study *Consumer Reports* did assessed 10 brands of ginseng. All 10 labels designated milligrams of ginseng per tablet, which were similar between brands but none of the labels had the amount of ginsenosides, thought to be the active ingredient. *Consumer Reports* analyzed all 10 brands and found the amount of ginsenosides varied from 0.6 mg to 23 mg.

So if a patient buys one brand because it is on sale or because the name is familiar, that patient may be getting 23 mg of ginsenocides in a 650 mg tablet. And ginseng is not one of the most benign herbs. It has estrogen-like effects and if patients are doing fine with one brand and then change to another, they may well think they have made no change because all they can see is that amount of ginseng on the label. But, indeed, they have made a significant change because in the next brand they may get only 0.6 mg of ginsenocides.

There have been more studies on variation of doses and the results are all over the map with herbal preparations. We tried to do a study on echinacea in our clinic and we went to Germany for echinacea. We had it analyzed in a lab at home and there wasn't any echinacea at all.

So, in summary, there is no guarantee that a plant's active ingredients are in a given pill or that dosages make sense and are in a bioavailable form. It is also not usually known what else is in the pill, whether the pills are safe, or that the next bottle will have the same ingredients in the same combination. In my mind, comparing FDA-regulated medications with herbal medication regulation is like comparing Word Perfect to Word Pretty Good.

Now to the sources of toxicity in the herbal medications themselves: first of all, there is some direct toxicity and I like to think of it as "plants aren't stupid." Darwin was right. There are evolutionary ways to protect oneself. If you are a plant, you don't want to be eaten. You make yourself toxic to the liver, and indeed one sees liver toxicity as a redundant theme. The other toxicity that seems to pop out all the time is interference with coagulation. In fact that's how warfarin is derived — from clover.

There are drug-supplement interactions and there are also supplement-supplement interactions. About the latter we have no idea. That's the biggest "black box." And then, with a lack of quality control, various adulterants may be present.

Drug-herbal interactions are fairly easy to predict if one knows the mechanism of action of the herb. For example, we know that licorice has aldosterone-like effects, so it makes sense that it will affect potassium loss and decrease the effect of spirolactone in antihypertensives. We know that black cohosh is a plant containing estrogen, and it will increase the effect of any therapeutically prescribed estrogens.

Most work recently has been done with St. John's Wort, showing that it decreases the metabolism of theophylline, highly active antiretroviral treatments, and Coumadin. However, it is a mistake to tell your patient, "Quit taking that St. John's Wort because you are taking theophylline, too," If balance has been achieved between herbs and drugs, destabilizing it can have serious effects.

There are other instances in which effects go the other way. For instance, NSAIDs can actually decrease the efficacy of feverfew, if feverfew is being used for migraines and NSAIDs are being used for migraines as well.

I think the clinician needs to have a ready reference. The one I like to support is *The Natural Pharmacist: Natural Health Bible from the Most Trusted Alternative Health Site in the World (Your A-Z Guide to Over 300 Conditions, Herbs, Vitamins, and Supplements)* by Steven Bratman, M.D. and David Kroll, Ph.D. It's written for lay people, but it is excellently referenced. General Nutrition's website (www.gnc.com) is straightforward and nonbiased. They give cautions about herbs not to use, contraindications, and some studies about efficacy as well. Other good and reliable sources are 1-800-MEDWATCH and www.fda.gov.

Reporting of possible adverse interactions is basically anecdotal, but without postmarketing surveillance, that is what there is to rely on. So if a patient wants to use an herb, I am likely to condone it if it is generally accepted as safe, if he is not taking a lot of other medications and if it is indicated for the problem.

What studies of chiropractic do we have? In a study done in Sweden, 625 patients from 10 different practices, with a total of 858 visits, were assessed. It was found that there were side effects, but that they were benign and self-limited: primarily limited to local discomfort, pain, fatigue, and headache, and more common at the start of treatment. Side effects tended to go away as treatments were continued.

In Norway, a study was done in 1997 with 100 chiropractic doctors, 1,052 new patients and more than 4,000 treatments. 55 percent of patients said they had at least one reaction over their six treatments, but 85 percent of these were rated as mild-to-moderate.

A retrospective study in Denmark found an estimate of one stroke for every 1.3 million cervical treatments. In the only American analysis I could find, a retrospective study done in 1996 in California asked neurologists how many patients they had seen in the last two years who experienced neurologic complications within 24 hours of seeing a chiropractor. Recall bias is a serious problem and it tells nothing about the end of chiropractic treatments, but they did come up with 55 strokes, 60 myelopathies and 30 radiculopathies from the 177 of 486 neurologists who responded. Some of the case reports in the literature describe head and neck complications, arterial hematomas, and emboli, but give no idea about the frequency.

Moving on to acupuncture, the first prospective study I found was from Japan with 55,000 patients, with only 64 events reported — however they asked the practitioners to report the events. In Germany, in a much smaller study, 29 percent of patients reported at least one event, with events occurring in 9 percent of all the treatments.

Another Japanese study revealed that there was an increased risk of hepatitis C with a history of acupuncture use. It's incredibly important to tell patients that practitioners should only use disposable needles.

From the case reports, by far the most common adverse events are associated with acupuncture pain and vagal reactions, and then hypotension and angina, because of the vagal reactions. Other complications are fairly rare; but infection, bleeding, dermatitis, edema, nerve injury and retained needles have been reported. If one mixes acupuncture with other therapies, anticoagulation patients should be excluded. There has been a recommendation by the Licensing Bureau of Acupuncturists that urges that therapists be trained in basic CPR skills.

For massage adverse events, there are no studies. The case reports are fairly interesting to read but do not give an idea of frequency, They include hepatic hematoma, urethral stent displacement, renal artery embolization, hearing loss, carotid artery dissection, destructive thyrotoxicosis, and fluid shifts in edematous patients.

I met with biofeedback practitioners I work with and told them I couldn't find anything about safety of biofeedback when mixed with conventional treatments. They claimed it to be effective for reducing blood pressure and perhaps in diabetes, too.

Colonic enemas are based on the theory that one must clean out the colon. I guess people don't realize it but the colon cleans itself out and you have a total replacement of the colonic lining every three days. If you want to do it this way, what's used is hypotonic solutions like coffee and water and massive fluid shifts can occur.

The safe-versus-unsafe concept for busy clinicians is very important. I think if we are going to teach physicians about alternative medicine, we have to listen to Hippocrates and, "first, do no harm." Therapies that routinely have a higher risk of being unsafe, I advise against. Interventions that tend to be safe, I condone and sometimes recommend. With supplements that cannot really be labeled as safe or unsafe, one needs to use a good reference and hope that there's better reporting. But I come back to a central theme; do not alienate patients. Work with them. Figure out why they want the treatment. Maybe there is something you can offer them.

What Physicians Need to Know About Medicinal Herbs

Lenore Arab, Ph.D.
University of North Carolina at Chapel Hill

As a nutritionist, I think that any parts of plants that we may eat, whether as teas or substance or supplements, are nutrition. As an epidemiologist, I see a tremendous need to capture the natural experiment that is going on: to assess the safety and efficacy of substances that people are self-prescribing for many different reasons, in amounts and frequencies that we wouldn't be allowed to test in clinical trials.

Part of my concern in this area is that there are groups of patients, such as cancer survivors, who are taking substances that can actually be harmful. As a cancer epidemiologist, I think there is a tremendous difference between what we should be doing to prevent cancer and what we might be doing to prevent the growth of tumors. We've seen some very important examples: the beta carotene trials were very informative and very disappointing.

Medicinal efficacy for herb use is prevalent and growing. Half of all alternative therapies are either medical herb use or massage. Real risks are involved in the use of both and there are also proven benefits. This presentation deals with why we need to teach about herbs, what we need to teach, and how we should be teaching.

The incorporation of medicinal herbs into medical treatment in western civilization began with Paracelsus who gave us that wonderful phrase, "The dose determines the poison." He became medical director in Basel and was driven out because of his alternative approaches, which according to Stedman's were a "a strange mixture of conceit, showmanship, senseless bombast, mysticism, astrology and sound medical wisdom."

Physicians need to know about use of medicinal herbs for several reasons. For example, some medical herbs can interfere with surgery and with prescribed medications. There are problems with bleeding in people who are taking high doses of ginseng. Antioxidants may interfere with chemotherapy.

What can we teach about unproven remedies? At a recent meeting experts were asked to comment about the efficacy and safety of

214

particular herbs. The group considered the use of saw palmetto for benign prostatic hypertrophy to be proven for short term, but not long-term use. St. John's Wort was held to be promising; ginseng as unproven. Gingko was regarded as useful in alleviating dementia but to be without effect in healthy individuals. The use of comfrey was considered to be unproven; so was garlic.

More is known about safety than about efficacy but probably not enough. Side effects from saw palmetto are mild and infrequent; St. John's Wort may be associated with photosensitivity, mania and drug interactions. For ginseng: GI symptoms, nervousness, confusion, depression and neonatal effects have been reported. No serious adverse side effects have been reported for ginkgo. Although comfrey has proven to be hepatoxic, it is still used in salads and is available in health food stores. Garlic, in the doses usually consumed in foods, causes no serious adverse effects. In contrast, many side effects have been reported for echinacea, including anaphylactic reaction, dizziness and a drop in blood pressure.

Clinical trials of safety and efficacy of medicinal herbs are sorely needed along with pharmaceutical studies to identify and under-stand their active ingredients. Unfortunately, it is not likely that this information will be forthcoming soon enough to satisfy public health needs. At present, it is important to instruct physicians about the limits of knowledge about these substances.

Physicians need to know what to ask about the use of medicinal herbs, how to ask about what the patient is taking, and how to ask about and interpret patterns of usage and dosages. Unfortunately, obtaining details may be very complicated.

It is important that physicians not only learn what is known but also what is not known about popular medicinal herbs. They have to be able to say with assurance what has not yet been tested or what has been tested and shown to be ineffective. That applies not only to supplements. Many of these substances are creeping into the food supply in all kinds of ways, as teas and other foods, or as fortifications. These patient practices call for increased awareness about multiple sources by which medicinal herbs can enter the body.

Physicians need to know how to access reliable information. This cannot be provided in a one-hour class on herbalism. For example,

TABLE 1.

Some Herbs Used for
Benign Prostastic Hyperplagia

- Serenoa repens   (Saw Palmetto)

- Hyposis roopert   (S African Star Grass)

- Secale cereale   (Rye Grass Pollen)

- Pygeum africanu   (African Plum Tree)

- Urtica dioca   (Stinging Nettle)

- Curcubita pepo   (Pumpkin Seed)

a number of herbs other than saw palmetto are being used around the world for benign prostatic hypertrophy. These are indicated in (Table 1). All are in use, and some have been subjected to clinical trials (Table 2). In general, the evidence for their usefulness is insufficient and inconclusive. However, physicians need to know where they can access relevant information about adverse reactions and interactions associated with the use of such substances.

Physicians need also to be familiar with principles of toxicology. Recently, the National Academy of Sciences has begun to set upper safety limits for intake of nutrients. This information, and the theory behind it, should be transmitted. Knowledge about "dangerous" herbs that are in widespread use, as well as interactions, need to be second nature to physicians. To summarize the current status of the knowledge base about herbal medications: there are scant epidemiological data, very few clinical trials and almost no information about interactions.

Physicians also need to know about nutrient supplements that are being taken by the same people who are taking high doses of medicinal herbs. That number is large: about half the population, according the NHANES III data. They have to be aware of the new

TABLE 2.

Clinical Trials for Herbs Used for Benign Prostastic Hyperplagia

■ Serenoa repens	19 trials, n=2939
■ Hyposis roopert	4 studies, 519 men
■ Secale cereale	4 trials 163 men
■ Pygeum africanu	12 trials, 717 men
■ Urtica dioca	5 trials, 543 men
■ Curcubita pepo	1 study, 55 men

standards for recommended intake, including the upper limits, and that multiple mega doses of nutrients can add up. One example is the use of high doses of Tums.

Extremely important is understanding that substances that are quite innocuous in general may not be safe for vulnerable groups. Some of the vulnerable individuals have preexisting conditions; others may absorb the products of herbal medications with unusual rapidity. Some, such as women who are pregnant or lactating, may run into problems because of other medications.

In summary, all physicians should learn the basics of commonly used herbs and how to access reliable information on the spectrum of herbs that are in current usage. They have to be aware of the current limits of knowledge in order to feel confident about the information they are delivering, including drug interactions and safety. Instruction about herbal medications should be provided not in special classes on alternative medicines but side-by-side with accredited therapies. For example, with respect to benign prostatic hypertrophy, there should not be one course that deals with tradition therapies and another that deals with alternative therapies; rather, both should be considered concurrently. Physicians should not separate the world of medicine into alternative and conventional: both should be taught in the same context.

As to how to gain the needed information, there are many alternatives and approaches. Among these are international meetings on medicinal herbs, videotapes of scientific reviews, monographs on safety and efficacy, meta-analyses of effects, and web-based courses. We need to help in this regard by creating reliable web sites that contain adequate information on actions/interactions, risk groups, and provide guidance and navigation to other reputable sites for more detailed information. And then, we need to make sure the information that is out there is kept current.

Section V
Professional and Research Issues/Consensus and Recommendations

Complementary/Alternative Medicine in the Making of a Physician and Other Health Care Professionals

Michael Whitcomb, M.D.
Association of American Medical Colleges

What I thought would be most useful is to provide a framework that would serve as a point of reference as you consider recommendations. Specifically, I want to do four things:

— I want to share with you the perspective of the Association of American Medical Colleges on this issue since much discussion has been directed to what it is that medical schools should do and what it is that we, as an organization in which medical schools are members, have been doing to try to focus the attention of schools on issues related to CAM.

— I want to present some general educational goals which I think are consistent with the association's position.

— I also want to discuss the dynamics of curriculum change. As you think about recommendations, it is very important to have a context and to not overreach, because overreaching tends to lead to outright dismissal of recommendations.

— And I want to begin with a statement of the way that we view education theory.

My responsibilities at the AAMC are basically for medical education. As we think about how we work with our members, we try to have some guiding principles that govern us. The association, in the development of its strategic plan of a few years ago, identified certain principles to guide us as we do our daily work.

One of those is that the AAMC should stimulate changes in medical education to create a better alignment of educational content and goals with evolving societal needs, practice patterns and scientific developments. I spend my time in pursuit of that particular commitment, and therefore get to visit medical schools a lot. We work with curriculum committees and education deans, clerkship directors and course directors. All of it is related to change, trying to bring a national perspective to what are often considered internal issues.

I think these can be dealt with better if people understand there are national perspectives and that in fact, there is a context for what a given dean may be suggesting.

We start from the following: What is the purpose of medical education? We suggest that the purpose is to prepare physicians to meet what have been defined as the goals of medicine. I am talking about the biomedical model. Therefore, the responsibility of those individuals who have the responsibility within institutions for the design and conduct of educational programs is to provide opportunities, within the context of those programs, for learners to acquire the knowledge, the skills and the attitudes that they need for the practice of medicine.

In modern life, that means for practice of a specialty of medicine. It is important to understand that reality as one begins to think about how to plan a continuum of education. The medical student education program is not intended to prepare students for the practice of medicine in the most immediate future. It is to prepare students with a general professional education. It should provide a foundation which is appropriate for all physicians to build upon as they continue learning through the formal parts of their education, graduate medical education, residencies and as life-long learners.

Residency should reinforce and expand on that. If one thinks about the education of doctors, almost all discussion has been on the curriculum, but that's not the way we educate doctors. We educate doctors across the continuum.

And so, the question before us is: what's the relevance of CAM to the practice of medicine? If it has no relevance, there is no reason that it should be in the curriculum or in residency programs. But if it has relevance, then we have a responsibility to make sure that there are opportunities for students and for learners at the resident level to acquire whatever knowledge, skills and attitudes are needed for them to be able to practice effectively.

A couple of years ago the association published a document, which is in many respects a consensus document, which took a stab at defining what we believe that a physician should be. Like all consensus documents there is language that may be too general, but it does provide a framework for thinking about education. It also gives some insight into the way that the medical education community views this issue, or at least viewed it a few years ago.

This document was distributed to the dean and the associate dean of every medical school in the United States and Canada. In a number of schools it was shared with curriculum committees or others. If we are going to make recommendations about education programs, we have to have some vision, some understanding of what a physician is to be. I think one of the very important points is that medicine is evolutionary and, therefore, educational programs must be evolutionary. That document talks about physicians, not about medical students. It says:

— Doctors, in their interactions with patients, must seek to understand the meaning of patient's stories in the context of the patient's belief and family and cultural values.

— They must avoid being judgmental when the patient's beliefs and values conflict with their own.

— They must engage in life-long learning to remain current in their understanding of the scientific basis of medicine.

— They must understand the scientific basis and evidence of effectiveness for each of the therapeutic options that are available for patients at different times in the course of the patient's condition, and be prepared to discuss those options with patients in an honest and objective fashion.

— They must be sufficiently knowledgeable of both traditional and nontraditional modes of care to provide intelligent guidance to their patients.

— They must acknowledge and respect the roles of other health professionals in providing needed services to individual patient populations or communities.

That's a large framing context. So, having reached a consensus articulating that, what does that mean for our purpose here? And what has the association done in pursuit of that?

First of all, in that statement we said that we are not resistant to the notion that nontraditional approaches to treatment have a role to play in thinking about the responsibility of physicians. The association is an organization which does its business in many ways, but fundamentally it tries to bring together members of our communities to work on issues of importance across the various missions of academic medical centers. Within that, there is the Group on Educational Affairs which involves the associate deans for education at every level and facility. It is the largest medical education group in the world with over 3,500 individual members.

The annual meeting of the association is largely a meeting of the Group on Educational Affairs, and there has been for the past few years a special interest group on CAM. The purpose of that is to bring together people to talk about the kinds of model programs that we might think about and share with others within the community whose interests might be in other aspects of education, in order to make sure that this view is represented.

At the spring meeting this past year, the keynote speaker was Dr. Andrew Weil who came to share his views on this issue. There was a plenary session devoted to CAM. Steve Strauss from the NIH was one of the speakers, and medical schools had an opportunity to discuss what they were doing. I think you might be surprised that the great majority of medical schools are currently involved in activities related to the introduction of CAM-relevant content into the curriculum. It is farther advanced in some schools than in others, but there is no resistance to the idea that this content ought to be part of the educational perspective and that it ought to be part of the general foundation provided for medical students.

I hope I have convinced you that AAMC is not hostile to the concept. The question really gets down to what is appropriate and what is inappropriate. Let me share with you what I believe is appropriate as it relates to educational goals for medical students:

— First, students have to understand that a large percentage of individuals who seek the care of physicians are also seeking the care of non-physician providers.

— They need to understand that the therapies that are being

prescribed by those practitioners are therapies that may be efficacious in some cases. They also may be harmful. They may be harmful in and of themselves, or they may be harmful because of interactions with therapies prescribed by physicians.

— They need to understand that some of those individuals who seek their help will be uncomfortable and unwilling to tell them that they are involved in therapy prescribed by non-physicians.

— And they need to begin to develop skills that would allow them to create a doctor/patient relationship in which patients will feel safe to reveal the fact that they are also under the care of a non-physician, and that they are able, in a very safe way, to have a discussion with a patient about such care and to be able to provide their own guidance.

That's what I think medical students need to learn. I do not think they need to learn a list of herbs. I do not think that they need to learn how to do spinal manipulation. Again, I want to emphasize that the purpose of the medical student educational program is to provide a foundation. To varying degrees, the specifics will be more relevant to physician practitioners in one specialty than another and one can begin to differentiate that knowledge as one goes on.

Let me talk about curriculum change dynamics to make several points. In the United States, the higher education curriculum is the prerogative of the faculty. We may wish it were not the case, but it is, and there is, therefore, a process that has to be engaged in to build consensus among the faculty in whatever governing mechanisms exist. They vary tremendously across 125 schools.

It's also important to understand that, unlike what many people think, content in the curriculum in educational experiences generally should not be viewed as a change agent. Long study of medical education in this country shows that when something has a level of acceptance within the medical education community, it begins to appear within educational programs. If there is no acceptance in the community, how would one construct educational programs that have meaning for the physician?

In short, focusing on courses or on hours in the context of the changes that occur in the structure of the medical school curriculum is a misplaced effort. Medical school curricula are going through a process in which there is a shift from individual, departmentally-owned courses to courses which are integrated across the curriculum and taught by multi-disciplinary teams. Therefore, asking if one has a course on CAM doesn't mean, if the answer is no, that there isn't appropriate content in the curriculum.

And, to emphasize a point I keep making, not everything that a doctor needs to know has to be in the medical school curriculum, though there's a tendency to think that's what we have to do. Too, curricula will always evolve, so what may be today should not be viewed as what will necessarily be tomorrow.

The final point I want to make has to do with educational methodologies. Medical schools will approach the introduction of content that the faculty view as appropriate and the design of educational experiences based upon the resources of the individual institutions. There is no one way to say that this must be done. We have curricula which are largely case-based and problem-based. We have curricula that are fully integrated across four years. There are all kinds of curricula in medical schools in this country. The issue is not a course. It's not that you must have a standardized patient. It is the responsibility of the faculty, given the resources that are available, to determine how best to meet the responsibilities that they have to their students.

Having made a judgment that certain content is relevant and certain education experiences are appropriate, how does one do that? One of the big challenges in many schools is the resource of faculty. If existing faculty are not engaged in that activity — as is true in many of the contemporary topics confronting medical education — then one has the challenge of figuring out where to find people who can provide knowledgeable instruction. That can be achieved through collaborative arrangements with other schools; or it may best be accomplished through web-based technology applications that can serve students wherever they may be.

Highlights of Discussion Sessions

A lively discussion centered around the extent to which CAM therapies entailed placebo effects. Part of the discussion dealt with "old-style" medical education, an essential ingredient of which was apprenticeship to a caring physician in a caring environment.

CAM providers don't interpret their results in terms of a placebo but prefer to deal in self-healing. Their work comes from a tradition that believes in the ability of the body to heal itself and starts with a philosophy that, if you believe the body has the ability to heal, then the goal of physicians and healers is to facilitate that process.

One participant described a course at the University of Arizona called "the art of medicine." In the course, students discuss topics such as the rationale for listening to patients and the power of suggestion. Students are then put in a clinical situation to practice what they have learned, while psychologists observe and provide feedback about communication skills and their relationships to patients. Cases are discussed in the context of patient belief systems which are used as a foundation for developing treatment plans. Students also experience, as patients, alternative therapies as well as psychoanalytic therapies.

Another participant reinforced the effectiveness of direct experience as a teaching tool, describing how students or residents who were there to observe were either hypnotized or hooked up for biofeedback when patients failed to show up for scheduled appointments. Through biofeedback, for instance, they were able to see that by altering their thinking they could change body responses. Such experiences led students to become more interested in CAM approaches.

Another theme of the discussion highlighted some of the salient points related to the education of young physicians made during discussion sessions and, at the same time, reflect the varied perspectives offered by participants. With representatives from both academic medicine and a number of CAM disciplines participating, discussion sessions during the conference reflected the diverse points of view around the table—as planners had intended. Despite their different perspectives, though, participants were able to identify many of the difficult questions that surround the issue of what medical students ought to know about complementary and alternative medicine, or CAM. They also made a number of observations and suggestions that helped the group formulate a set of recommendations to address those questions. Those recommendations are included at the end of the Chairman's Summary (page 25).

As their discussions progressed, participants agreed that there is no specific entity that is CAM, for CAM encompasses a range of therapies and approaches to healing, some of which can be and some have been—scientifically validated while others are supported mainly by anecdotal reports and testimonials. They acknowledged the need to identify those which may be beneficial, those which can be harmful and those which are more benign. In essence, each modality should be evaluated with respect to risk versus benefit.

Against this varied backdrop, the debate over what physicians should know about CAM led participants from academic medicine to call for rigorous testing of CAM practices according to Western scientific standards, whereas others suggested that testing to meet the double-blind, controlled trial "gold standard" of Western medicine would be superfluous for practices that are already in wide use and have proven over centuries to be benign.

Yet, it was agreed physicians need to be aware of a full range of CAM practices so they can answer patient questions and alert their patients to CAM practices that might be beneficial or harmful and those that would, at least, do no harm. Where appropriate, they might refer them to qualified CAM practitioners. The participants agreed that familiarity with CAM practices could contribute to cultural awareness, the caring aspects of medicine and to professionalism in medicine. Physicians especially need to know about supplements and herbal remedies because of the potential for interaction with prescription medications, just as CAM practitioners need to recognize when a patient should be referred to a physician and how herbal remedies interact with and affect many prescription medicines.

Participants from academic medicine observed that the challenge of introducing CAM is part of the larger problem of how to introduce any new material to already overcrowded curricula. Physicians do not need to know the specifics of whole CAM systems, such as Chinese medicine or ayurveda, but they do need to know what these systems involve, information that can be—and in many situations already is being—integrated into existing courses.

But before deciding how much and in what form CAM should be added to medical curricula, one participant suggested that a "reasoned assessment" should be made of what a physician is supposed to be in 20 years. Over the course of years, nurses, physician assistants and other health professionals have taken over many of the responsibilities that once belonged only to physicians. These range from such activities as physical and occupational therapy to prescribing infant formulas and taking blood pressures.

Recognizing that other health professionals have assumed responsibilities and activities previously confined to the domain of the physician, care must be taken not to go the other direction with CAM by transferring to future physicians skills and a knowledge base that overlaps with those which other practitioners already possess, one participant warned.

Efforts to introduce information about CAM to medical education now come at a particularly awkward time for the medical profession, for managed care has imposed time constraints on physician-patient contact time and financial strictures have caused physicians to operate at a financial disadvantage. Not only has this has meant spending less time with individual patients but academic health centers have stripped themselves to the point where real people don't answer phones, staffs have been cut to the bone, and patients wait unreasonable lengths of time for appointments. The idea that physicians should be trained in a way that encourages them to spend more time with patients—as CAM providers are said to do—is directly contrary to what is happening in the real world.

A number of participants emphasized the need to encourage the two sides to move beyond their current confrontational need to denounce each other and focus instead on identifying those CAM practices that are valuable. The report that people see CAM providers more often than they see primary care providers does not necessarily mean that what these CAM providers offer is more valuable, but it does suggest Western scientific medicine is not satisfying completely patient needs and focusing on the importance of exploring what is happening in health care and of understanding what providers on both sides are, or are not, providing to their patients.

One participant observed that people are turning to CAM not because they are disillusioned with conventional medicine but because they want to explore all their options and to draw upon more than one way of thinking. This is particularly true of "baby boomers," the seriously ill and those who find insufficient relief from chronic illness from western medicine. Indeed, another pointed out, western medicine is spreading throughout the world because it has proven so powerful for dealing with many acute conditions and diseases; however, it is not as effective in chronic illnesses. This suggests people are not running from western medicine when they go to a CAM provider but are seeking what medicine is not providing in terms of time, healing and care.

A number of comments explored ways the two sides could learn from each other with repeated emphasis on the need for rigorous scientific testing of promising CAM therapies to satisfy the public "need-to-know" and to assess risk: benefit relationships. Historically, the scientific approach has demystified western medicine, which is constantly evolving in response to new research and new approaches to treatment. Consequently, practitioners are now more subject to analysis and scrutiny by both their colleagues and the public. If CAM practices were subjected to more rigorous testing, they, too, would undergo the same kind of evolution—and be subject to more analysis and scrutiny.

Considerable discussion emphasized issues of cultural diversity. One participant noted that physicians need to acknowledge and understand cultural differences, for they account for different ways of seeing the same symptoms and the same illnesses. One example cited of why this is important was the experience of a Hmong family that did not consider epilepsy a disease; the family resisted medical treatment and relied instead on the healing powers of religious belief. In such instances, medical management may save a life but must take into account that success entails the risk of contaminating and isolating that person from a culture.

The ability to respect cultural differences is essential, but how far should it go? A number of participants asked that, raising a number of problems that "hover at the fringe" of diversity and cultural differences. For instance, people from most cultures want vaccinations, antibiotics and surgery when needed and usually these services are covered by insurance. But what happens if a patient is a Navajo who wants a healing ceremony with a Navajo medicine man in addition to western medical care? Should health insurance also pay for the healing ceremony? What happens about differences in belief that jeopardize the lives of others or management that is diametrically opposite medical practices? One example offered was the folk belief in many parts of the world that a child with diarrhea should have no oral intake, including fluids, in order to "rest" the bowel, a belief that has contributed to countless childhood deaths that could have been prevented by oral rehydration therapy.

The need for medical students to learn to take the time to develop a relationship and learn to communicate with patients who have a different belief system was emphasized. At the same time, students need to learn that overcoming differences will not be easy. Will majority medical students be able to learn about folk practices and then be able to communicate their understanding to patients? Will majority physicians be able to get patients from different backgrounds to follow a medical regimen that may be contrary to different belief systems? Such questions underscore the need for physicians to develop cultural awareness, to understand where their patients come from and what the patient brings to the encounter. Physicians need to understand, and be alert to, the impact on their patients of having sons in jail, teen-age daughters who have children, working two or three jobs, or not having enough money to pay the rent and put food on the table.

In the specific context of patient/physician communication, discussion emphasized the point that health care providers need not only to be aware of and sensitized to feelings of shame and humiliation, but also to understand how to deal with these feelings. To one participant, this need underscored the importance of good communication and not making assumptions about why patients have come, to understand the needs of their patients and to focus on the cultural background. They should not simply assume they understand the patient's problem. By listening carefully and then asking "how are you hoping I could help you?" a student can learn to identify the patient's main priority and can then start negotiating. Too often, students today do not learn to ask this simple question and inadvertently humiliate the patient. If they fail to understand why the patient is really there—which often has nothing to do with the physician's assumptions—any chance for a meaningful encounter has ended.

Physicians are themselves subjected to shame and humiliation from their earliest student days to their current practices. Today, even a call from a patient care office carries with it a threat. But physicians need to realize the patients' humiliation also. For example, at the start of every encounter with the medical establishment, patients are questioned about their financial status and insurance coverage, and then are left waiting until someone finally gets around to seeing them.

In discussion about specific CAM interventions, participants focused on potential safety problems with different therapies. By law, the Food and Drug Administration can remove supplements and herbal products from the market only for reasons of safety or lack of efficacy. As a practical matter, the agency rarely exercises this authority for a number of reasons, among them lack of resources and congressional constraints on taking any action without absolute proof of unsafety, which is difficult to achieve.

It was noted that herbal remedies and supplements, which can be found in almost any grocery store, are widely taken because people believe that "natural" equals "safe". One participant emphasized that the safety of CAM practices must be judged on a case-by-case basis. Too, it is important to recognize that while active ingredients in medicines can be identified with great precision, there is no such assurance with herbal remedies where there can be huge variability. People take whatever comes in the box without knowing what's in that box. With many of these supplements, it is not clear whether an active ingredient or some other ingredient accounts for any activity, though a great deal of research is being done to answer the question of whether an ingredient alone is active or whether an interaction is responsible.

The idea of trying to find a single active ingredient is based on the assumption that there is a single ingredient that will work when removed from a plant matrix but, as one participant reminded, the experience with beta carotene challenged that assumption. Whether such questions will ever be resolved is not clear. It costs as much as 350 million dollars to identify an active ingredient and then take a product through the kinds of trials required for FDA approval. Since companies can't patent a product but can only patent an extraction process—which makes it difficult to recoup such an investment—there's little financial incentive to answer this kind of question.

It was also pointed out that herbal products can not be standardized unless an active ingredient is identified. Even if the active ingredient is standardized so that it can be tested, there is no way of knowing what other ingredients are doing, whether they are the sources of any toxicities or beneficial actions.

Another participant warned that patients need to learn to look for "red flags" when evaluating CAM practices and practitioners. This involves asking about training, the effectiveness of treatments, risks and benefits. Any promise of a cure 100 percent of the time or no risks should be an automatic "red flag.

A recurrent theme through the discussions was the need for information about herbal products, their effects and interactions. This information should be readily available to students, physicians and CAM providers as well as their patients. Web sites that are reliable and constantly updated fill this need.

Physicians need to know as much about herbal remedies as they do about drugs, one participant emphasized, because herbs are drugs. The danger with herbal remedies is that patients are self-prescribing in doses they don't know, responding to advertising that assures a product is safe and 100 percent effective. Physicians need to know what their patients are taking because these remedies can affect medications the physician prescribes. They also need to know about these remedies to at least keep up with patients because so many already know about herbal alternatives before they go to a physician.

On the other side, CAM practitioners also need to know about drugs, their manifestations and the ways different drugs interact with different herbs and with medications that their patients are taking. More and more reports are appearing of toxic interactions between herbal ingredients and prescribed medications

Finally, in the discussion of curriculum change in medical education, one participant suggested that the issue of introducing CAM is not one of identifying how many hours or precisely what should be taught but to teach medical students how to evaluate all therapies—including those that come from biomedical science.

Another pointed out that clinical education is no longer dominated by senior experienced medical educators and physicians as role models. Instead, exposure to medical care is largely via junior physicians in a hospital setting. This is changing. CAM principles of practice can help in alleviating this shortcoming.

Most participants agreed on the need to teach students to listen, to reach out to patients and to have an empathetic response. But with the extraordinary pace of change, the rapid introduction of new technology and the increasing pressures to deliver cost-effective medicine, they wondered how this could be achieved. While some systems of medical training emphasize communication skills and helping students develop their sensitivities—Tibetan medicine was offered as an example— it is not clear how this could be implemented in western medicine.

Several participants noted that, in addition to a chronic lack of resources, the real roadblock is the faculty, since few faculty members have any familiarity with CAM theories or practices. One suggestion offered for overcoming this problem included identifying specific faculty members who can take responsibility for introducing a subject; another suggestion was the organizing of workshops on CAM for faculty members.

The annual AAMC survey of new medical school graduates shows that almost two thirds of those who respond—and, it was reported, response is high—believe their education about CAM has been inadequate. Schools are gradually adding CAM to curriculum content but this change is taking place school-by-school, in different ways and in different degrees. Thus the topic of this conference was timely, and the need to grapple with the issues raised will remain for the forseeable future.

Editor: Mary Hager
Design and production: Klaboe Design, New York
Cover design/photomontage: David Klaboe
Cover photos: corbisimages.com. & David Klaboe
Conference photos: pp. 8, 14, 15: Scott Mitchell
Printed in USA by Cinnamon Graphics, Inc., New York